Lippincott's  Magnetic Resonance Imaging Review

G000092940

Gregory L. Wheeler, BS, RT(R) (MR)
Gregory L. Wheeler and Associates
Oakland, California
and GPW Medical Imaging Consultants
San Francisco, California

Kathryn E. Withers, RT(R) (MR)
New Hanover Hospital
Wilmington, North Carolina

Acquisition Editor: Andrew Allen
Coordinating Editorial Assistant: Patty Moore
Compositor: Richard G. Hartley
Printer/Binder: R. R. Donnelley & Sons Company

Printed in the United States of America. For information write
Lippincott-Raven Publishers, 227 East Washington Square,
Philadelphia, Pennsylvania 19106-3780.

6   5   4   3   2   1

0-397-55156-8

Any procedure or practice described in this book should be applied by the
health care practitioner under appropriate supervision in accordance with
professional standards of care used with regard to the unique circumstances
that apply in each practice situation. Care has been taken to confirm the ac-
curacy of information presented and to describe generally accepted prac-
tices. However, the authors, editors, and publisher cannot accept any
responsibility for errors or omissions or for any consequences from application of the information in this book and make no warranty, express or im-
plied, with respect to the contents of the book. Every effort has been made
to ensure drug selections and dosages are in accordance with current recom-
mendations and practice.

Because of ongoing research, changes in government regulations, and the
constant flow of information on drug therapy, reactions, and interactions,
the reader is cautioned to check the package insert for each drug for indica-
tions, dosages, warnings, and precautions, particularly if the drug is new or
infrequently used.

Preface

This publication has been created to prepare technologists for the Advanced Level Examination in magnetic resonance imaging conducted by the American Registry of Radiologic Technologists (ARRT). Subsequent to the successful completion of the advanced level examination the letters (MR) (ARRT) will be added to your credentials.

There are 700 questions and answers in this review book. While the questions are not the exact questions that will be asked in the examination, they do follow the Content Specifications provided by the ARRT and are in a similar format to ones you will be asked. We recommend that you use this book as a review and as a study guide. It is designed to allow you to evaluate the content areas in which you are weak and provides additional references for you to gain additional knowledge. The questions vary in degree of difficulty and are meant to prepare and challenge the reader.

The MR advanced level examination contains 175 questions. The questions are divided into four sections as in the Content Specifications. We have provided four times the number of questions for each section. There are 525 questions in the beginning section of the book. There are also 175 additional post test questions which we recommend you use as a mock registry examination subsequent to answering the 525 questions. Each question has an answer with a short explanation and references for additional resources. There is also an appendix which includes the symbols and abbreviations used in this book.

To use the book we recommend that you first read each question and eliminate any answers that are obviously incorrect. Then begin to narrow the choices based on the wording of the question and the choices available. If you are unable to answer the question, circle the question and continue to the next one. You may find information in subsequent questions that will help you answer each of the questions asked. If you are still unable to answer the question, use the references for in-depth investigation.

While the primary goal of this project is to prepare you to take the advanced level examination we hope that it will be an excellent resource for your future MR educational needs.

Acknowledgments

I would like to offer sincere thanks to Robert Lufkin, MD, Associate Professor at the UCLA Medical Center and Karen L. Pary, RT, from the Academic Radiologists of Southern Illinois University for their excellent job reviewing the manuscript for this book. I would also like to thank Barry Noll and Jim Franklin for their constant support and assistance. Without their emotional support the project would not have been completed. I would like to acknowledge Mark Leszczynski for his support while completing this work. It is his constant prodding that gave me the drive. It is also important to acknowledge my co-author, Kate Withers, for her diligence during the long hours it took us to complete the book. Foremost, I would like to thank Divine Guidance for allowing me clarity of purpose and the will to succeed.

Gregory Wheeler

My dear family of eagles, Jay, Amy, and Aaron, have been a constant source of love, approval, and strength. Special thanks to our parents, Gloria, Jim, and Betty for all of the lessons on living life skillfully. I would like to thank Dr. Charles Williams for allowing me the opportunity to begin my journey in the realm of magnetic resonance imaging. Special thanks are sent to Bill Faulkner and Carolyn Kaut-Roth for their enormous contribution to our field through their seminars and publications. For the first time, technologists had information "on their level" which made it possible to gain a firm foundation on which to build. My appreciation to Mr. Edward Barnes of MTMI, a true entrepreneur, for his vision of educating technologists through his wonderful seminars. I would also like to thank Gregory Wheeler for his positive attitude, motivation, and class. He keeps me stretching. To my friend and colleagues at New Hanover Hospital, thank you for your kindness and support. And finally, I am thankful to the one who is my source of living water. Without Him, this life would be a desert.

Kate Withers

Table Of Contents

Patient Care and Safety

1. Select the purpose for patient screening.
   ____ a. explain the procedure/allay patient fears
   ____ b. acquire patient history
   ____ c. identify ferromagnetic materials within the patient
   ____ d. all of the above

2. Which of the following are exempt from basic screening procedures?
   ____ a. patient
   ____ b. accompanying family member
   ____ c. nursing staff/housekeeping
   ____ d. none of the above

3. If a patient states that 30 years ago, he had a small piece of metal removed from his eye, which method should be employed before scanning is to begin?
   ____ a. patient is OK to scan, after 30 years, scar tissue will hold any residual fragments in place
   ____ b. have your radiologist look at the patient's eye
   ____ c. plain films of the orbit
   ____ d. CT films of the orbit

4. Which of the following metals are probably ferrous?
   ____ a. nickel
   ____ b. cobalt
   ____ c. iron
   ____ d. all of the above

5. Which of the following cases would be safe to scan?
   ____ a. patient with an intracranial ferromagnetic aneurysm clip
   ____ b. patient with a thoracic aneurysm clip
   ____ c. patient with a known nonferrous intracranial aneurysm clip
   ____ d. b and c

6. Which of the following have been contraindicated for MRI scans?
   _____ a. prosthetic hip replacements
   _____ b. cochlear implants/Duraphase penile implant
   _____ c. Silastic heart valves
   _____ d. intravascular coils, filters, and stents

7. Which of the following patients should probably not be scanned?
   _____ a. patient with sickle cell anemia
   _____ b. patient in the 1st trimester of pregnancy
   _____ c. nursing mother
   _____ d. patient with high blood urea nitrogen level (BUN) and low creatine levels

8. Since the magnetic field may interfere with the operation of certain mechanical devices, which of the following have been FDA contraindicated for MRI scans?
   _____ a. neurostimulators
   _____ b. bone growth stimulators
   _____ c. implantable drug infusion pumps
   _____ d. all of the above

9. Which of the following patients should not be scanned?
   _____ a. Vietnam veteran with a 20-cm piece if shrapnel in the right popliteal area
   _____ b. 70-year-old gentleman with a fatio eyelid spring
   _____ c. patient with a residual epicardial pacing lead in his chest
   _____ d. all of the above

10. The pediatric patient should be given nothing by mouth (NPO) for at least _____ hours before administering sedation.
    _____ a. 1
    _____ b. 2
    _____ c. 4
    _____ d. 10

11. Contrast reactions occur in a very small amount of patients. _____ is the most commonly reported contrast reaction.

____ a. headache

____ b. nausea

____ c. bronchospasm

____ d. hypotension

12. In the event that a patient develops severe bronchospasms after the injection of contrast, which drug would probably be administered by the nurse or radiologist?

____ a. epinephrine

____ b. Benadryl

____ c. atropine

____ d. valium

13. According to The Safety Committee of the Society for Magnetic Resonance Imaging, which of the following patients should be visually and verbally monitored?

____ a. elderly patients with soft voices

____ b. cardiac patients

____ c. sedated and pediatric patients

____ d. all of the above

14. If a patient with COPD came into your department receiving 2 liters of oxygen and began to have difficulty breathing, which of the following is advisable?

____ a. elevate their feet

____ b. give them a drink of orange juice

____ c. increase the oxygen to at least 10 liters

____ d. stop the scan and call the nurse

15. Normal oxygen saturation levels should be about ____%.

____ a. 55-65

____ b. 65-75

____ c. 75-85

____ d. 95-100

16. The pulse rate should be about _____ beats per minute.
    ___ a. 60-100
    ___ b. 100-120
    ___ c. 125-130
    ___ d. 40-50

17. According to the FDA, a severe reaction to MR contrast is described as:
    ___ a. life threatening or permanently disabling
    ___ b. headaches and nausea
    ___ c. dysphasia
    ___ d. magnetic hemodynamic effects

18. Since the intensity of the static magnetic field falls off as the third power of the distance from the magnet, it is advisable to place monitoring devices approximately _____ feet from the opening of the bore on a 1.5 T magnet.
    ___ a. 3
    ___ b. 12
    ___ c. 4
    ___ d. 8

19. Which of the following magnets would pose the most concern in regard to ferromagnetic projectiles?
    ___ a. a permanent magnet
    ___ b. a resistive magnet
    ___ c. a low-field superconductive magnet
    ___ d. a high-field superconductive magnet

20. _____ is the most important aspect of providing a safe MRI environment.
    ___ a. screening
    ___ b. shielding
    ___ c. shimming
    ___ d. education

21. _____ may be employed around the scanner to reduce the magnetic fringe field.
  ___ a. A Faraday cage
  ___ b. A Fourier transform
  ___ c. Steel in the walls
  ___ d. Active shimming

22. As of 1992, there have been over 75 reported incidents of
burns to MR patients. Which of the following do not present the potential for burns to the patient?
  ___ a. pulse oximeter
  ___ b. surface coil cable
  ___ c. electrocardiograph wire
  ___ d. all of the above

23. The environmental temperature should be about
_____ for optimum operation of MRI systems.
  ___ a. 65-75° F
  ___ b. 45-60° F
  ___ c. 35-55° F
  ___ d. 35-55° C

24. In order to prevent spurious radiofrequency (RF) waves
from entering the scan room area, _____ is employed.
  ___ a. Faraday cage
  ___ b. Fourier transform
  ___ c. steel in the walls
  ___ d. active shimming

25. The MRI *exclusion zone* for patients with pacemakers,
neurostimulators, or other metallic implants is at
the_____ level.
  ___ a. 1 gauss (G)
  ___ b. 5 G
  ___ c. 15 G
  ___ d. 20 G

26. The MRI *safety zone* begins at the door of the scan room. On a 1.5 T magnet, which of the following may safely enter the scan room in the event of an emergency?
    ____ a. crash cart
    ____ b. typical oxygen tank
    ____ c. stethoscope
    ____ d. none of the above

27. The scanning environment should maintain a relative humidity of about _____ percent.
    ____ a. 50-70
    ____ b. 10-20
    ____ c. 25-45
    ____ d. less than 10

28. _____ is the sudden boil off of cryogens that causes the collapse of the magnetic field.
    ____ a. shimming
    ____ b. ramping down
    ____ c. a quench
    ____ d. none of the above

29. Sudden release of cryogens into the room may cause which of the following?
    ____ a. patient injury due to panic
    ____ b. frostbite and asphyxiation
    ____ c. rupture of the tympanic membrane
    ____ d. all of the above

30. The proper procedure for getting a patient out of the scan room during a quench involves:
    ____ a. keeping the patient's head elevated as high as possible in the room as you exit
    ____ b. getting as close to the floor as possible as you exit
    ____ c. calling the radiologist for his opinion
    ____ d. calling the code team and waiting for their arrival

31. Which of the following should not be injected with gadolinium contrast agents?
   ____ a. patients with sickle cell anemia
   ____ b. pregnant patients
   ____ c. nursing mothers
   ____ d. all of the above

32. Describe the proper placement of surface coil cables:
   ____ a. placed away from the patient, along the side of the bore of the magnet
   ____ b. looped in a neat circle away from the patient
   ____ c. placed away from the patient, under padding, running straight down the bore of the magnet
   ____ d. braided with other cables that are present in the bore

33. Which of the following are important precautions concerning contrast agents?
   ____ a. protect from light and cold
   ____ b. check the color and consistency of the material
   ____ c. draw up contrast just prior to injection
   ____ d. all of the above

34. Which of the following statements is incorrect regarding the use of a surface coil?
   ____ a. remove all unplugged surface coils from the bore of the magnet before scanning
   ____ b. keep the length of cable to a minimum
   ____ c. make sure to cross or loop cables if there are two or more present in the bore
   ____ d. do not use cables that are frayed

35. When positioning a surface coil on a patient, it is impor-
    tant to remember that you will acquire _____ if the
    coil is a long distance from the patient.
    ___ a. greater signal-to-noise ratio (SNR)
    ___ b. better resolution
    ___ c. lower SNR
    ___ d. lower resolution

36. If a patient's arm touches the side of the bore, which of
    the following may result?
    ___ a. patient burn
    ___ b. detuning of the magnet, causing degrading of
           the images
    ___ c. the magnet may be thrown into a linear mode
           that could increase the amount of RF deposition
    ___ d. all of the above

37. Which of the following is a false statement regarding pa-
    tient burns?
    ___ a. make sure that the patient's arms do not touch
           the respiratory belt
    ___ b. keep electrically conductive material from di-
           rectly contacting the patient's skin
    ___ c. use only devices that are electrically and mag-
           netically MR compatible
    ___ d. do not let patient's skin come in direct contact
           with a surface coil

38. During a clinical MR scan, the patient is exposed to
    _____ different types of electromagnetic radiation.
    ___ a. 1
    ___ b. 2
    ___ c. 3
    ___ d. 0

39. According to the most recent FDA regulations, there are no adverse effects from short-term exposure to magnets of the following field strengths.
    ____ a. .5 T
    ____ b. 1.5 T
    ____ c. up to 2 T
    ____ d. up to 4 T

40. In a static field, _____ has been observed. It is the result of blood (conductive fluid) flowing through a magnetic field.
    ____ a. magneto hydrodynamic effect
    ____ b. elevation of the T wave
    ____ c. magnetic hemodynamic effect
    ____ d. all of the above

41. The static magnetic field strength is measured in _____ at isocenter and _____ outside the bore of the magnet.
    ____ a. T/G
    ____ b. G per cm/T per cm
    ____ c. G/T
    ____ d. mT/T

42. The primary effects of exposure to RF radiation is relate to tissue heating resulting from energy absorption. The FDA has determined the tissue heating limit to be _____.
    ____ a. .4 w/kg
    ____ b. .04 w/kg
    ____ c. 4 w/kg
    ____ d. none of the above

43. The name given to the unit of RF absorption is _____.
    ____ a. sensitization rate
    ____ b. specific absorption rate (SAR)
    ____ c. specialized absorption rate
    ____ d. all of the above

44. RF fields should not cause a core body temperature to rise greater than _____ .

_____ a. 1°C

_____ b. 10°C

_____ c. 1°F

_____ d. .01°C

45. Research has found that RF absorption causes an increase in the body temperature to be different in various parts of the body. This heating results more on the _____ surface and less on the _____ surface.

_____ a. inferior/superior

_____ b. posterior/anterior

_____ c. external/internal

_____ d. medial/lateral

46. Which monitor records the patient heart rate?

_____ a. photoplethysmograph

_____ b. end-tidal CO_2 monitor

_____ c. respiratory belt

_____ d. sphygmomanometer

47. Another name for the blood pressure cuff is _____ .

_____ a. ventilator

_____ b. sphygmomanometer

_____ c. electrocardiogram

_____ d. capnometer

48. Which of the following organs have proven to be the most sensitive to elevated temperatures during MRI scanning, because they have reduced capabilities for heat dissipation?

_____ a. pituitary/adrenal

_____ b. testis/prostate

_____ c. testis/eye

_____ d. eye/cuticles

49. The most common complications from sedation and anesthesia are respiratory depression and upper airway obstruction. Therefore, it is important that these patients' respiratory functions are closely monitored. Which of the following machines should be employed to monitor respiratory levels in these patients?

    ____ a. sphygmomanometer

    ____ b. capnometer

    ____ c. respiratory belt

    ____ d. plastic cup placed on the patient's chest

50. The chief concern in dealing with static magnetic fields is that of _____.

    ____ a. "the missile effect" produced by ferromagnetic materials

    ____ b. tissue heating

    ____ c. cardiac effects

    ____ d. experiencing magnetophosphenes

51. The linear gradient alters the magnetic field by _____ G/cm.

    ____ a. 1

    ____ b. .1

    ____ c. .4

    ____ d. 4

52. It is necessary to bind gadolinium to a _____ in order to decrease its toxicity in the body.

    ____ a. kaolin

    ____ b. bentonite

    ____ c. chelate

    ____ d. all of the above

53. Gradient magnetic field strength is measured in
    _____ or _____.
    ____ a. mTm/G per cm
    ____ b. mT per cm/G per m
    ____ c. cm per T/m per G
    ____ d. cm per kg/G per m

54. Which anatomical plane is oriented 90° to midline and divides the head into front and back halves?
    ___ a. axial
    ___ b. coronal
    ___ c. sagittal
    ___ d. off axis oblique

55. Which layer of meninges is the hard, fibrous covering that adheres to the inner table of the skull?
    ___ a. dura mater
    ___ b. arachnoid
    ___ c. pia mater
    ___ d. none of the above

56. Enlarged subarachnoid spaces located particularly around the base of the brain are called _____.
    ___ a. ventricles
    ___ b. meninges
    ___ c. periosteum
    ___ d. cisterns

57. Dips or grooves between the superficial bulges on the surface of the cerebrum are called _____.
    ___ a. sulci
    ___ b. gyri
    ___ c. peduncles
    ___ d. fissures

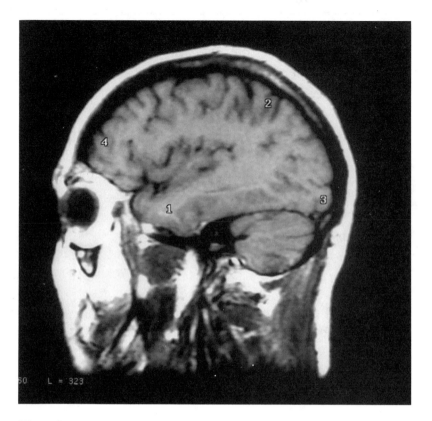

Figure 1

58. In Figure 1, arrow 1 is the _____ lobe of the cerebrum.

    ____ a. temporal

    ____ b. occipital

    ____ c. parietal

    ____ d. frontal

59. On Figure 1, the fissure that is located directly above the lobe on arrow 1 is called the _____ fissure.

    ____ a. sylvian

    ____ b. longitudinal

    ____ c. transverse

    ____ d. tentorial

60. The epithalamus, thalamus, and hypothalamus are considered the _____.

____ a. telencephalon

____ b. mesencephalon

____ c. diencephalon

____ d. all of the above

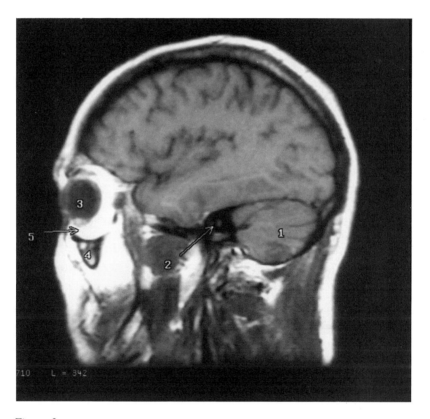

Figure 2

61. In figure 2, arrow 5 points to _____, which is a tissue that is bright on T1-weighted images.

____ a. fat

____ b. blood

____ c. hemosiderin

____ d. muscle

62. Identify arrow 2 in Figure 2.
    ___ a. the internal auditory canal (IAC)
    ___ b. the 7th and 8th nerves
    ___ c. the facial and vestibulocochlear nerves
    ___ d. all of the above

63. Which cranial nerve is considered the facial nerve?
    ___ a. III
    ___ b. VII
    ___ c. IX
    ___ d. VI

64. Which cranial nerve affects hearing and balance?
    ___ a. III
    ___ b. V
    ___ c. IX
    ___ d. VIII

65. Symptoms of a/an _____ include hearing loss, tinnitus, and dizziness.
    ___ a. acoustic neuroma
    ___ b. pituitary adenoma
    ___ c. glossopharyngeal neuroma
    ___ d. trigeminal neuralgia

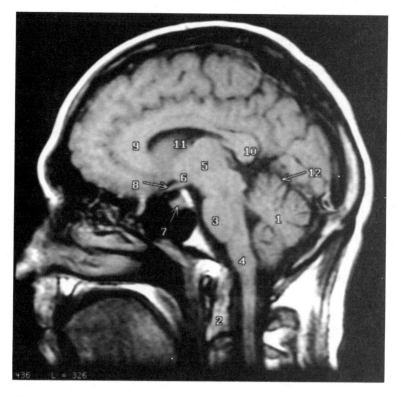

Figure 3

66. Identify the anatomy labeled 9 on Figure 3.
    ____ a. genu of the corpus callosum
    ____ b. splenium of the corpus callosum
    ____ c. fornix of the corpus callosum
    ____ d. body of the corpus callosum

67. Identify the structure labeled 3 on Figure 3.
    ____ a. midbrain
    ____ b. medulla
    ____ c. pons
    ____ d. thalamus

68. Identify the structure labeled 4 on Figure 3.

____ a. vermis

____ b. medulla

____ c. clivus

____ d. pons

69. The _____ is indicated by arrow 12 on Figure 3.

____ a. vermis

____ b. tentorium

____ c. cerebellar cistern

____ d. clivus

70. In Figure 3, structure 5 is a _____ structure.

____ a. muscular

____ b. glandular

____ c. white matter

____ d. gray matter

71. _____ is identified by arrow 8 on Figure 3.

____ a. pineal stalk

____ b. pituitary stalk

____ c. orbital fissure

____ d. optic chiasm

72. Identify 7 on Figure 3.

____ a. pituitary gland

____ b. pineal gland

____ c. sphenoid sinus

____ d. habenula

73. The anatomy identified by 3 on Figure 3 is part of the_____.

____ a. the cerebellum

____ b. the brain stem

____ c. the basal ganglia

____ d. the hypothalamus

74. _____ is a condition in which part of the cerebellar tonsil is displaced below the foramen magnum.
    ____ a. hydrocephalus
    ____ b. syringomyelia
    ____ c. Simmonds' disease
    ____ d. Chiari malformation

75. All of the following techniques should be employed except_____ when imaging the pituitary gland.
    ____ a. small field of view(FOV)
    ____ b. thin slices
    ____ c. increase in matrix
    ____ d. fat saturation

76. In order to differentiate a syrinx from a truncation artifact on a cervical spine scan, the technologist should employ which method?
    ____ a. enlarge the FOV or increase the matrix
    ____ b. put on inferior and superior saturation pulses
    ____ c. use gradient moment nulling
    ____ d. none of the above

77. In order to visualize the internal auditory canal, high resolution images are acquired in which planes?
    ____ a. axial and coronal
    ____ b. off axis oblique
    ____ c. sagittal and coronal
    ____ d. sagittal and axial

78. In order to visualize the pituitary gland, which planes are most useful?
    ____ a. axial and coronal
    ____ b. off axis oblique
    ____ c. sagittal and coronal
    ____ d. sagittal and axial

79. Describe the appearance of subacute intracranial hemor-
    rhage (greater than 7 days).

    ____ a. low signal on T1 and high signal on
             T2–weighted images
    ____ b. high signal on T1 and low signal on
             T2–weighted images
    ____ c. isointense on T1 and high signal on
             T2–weighted images
    ____ d. high signal on both T1– and T2–weighted im-
             ages

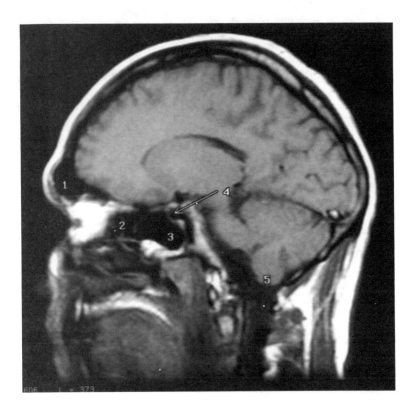

Figure 4

80. Number 2 in Figure 4 is the _____ sinus.

    ____ a. frontal
    ____ b. maxillary
    ____ c. ethmoid
    ____ d. sphenoid

81. In Figure 4, identify the structure marked 3.
    ___ a. frontal sinus
    ___ b. maxillary sinus
    ___ c. ethmoid sinus
    ___ d. sphenoid sinus

82. Identify the structure marked 1 in Figure 4.
    ___ a. frontal sinus
    ___ b. vermis
    ___ c. anterior cerebral artery
    ___ d. vertebral artery

83. Susceptibility effects are often apparent in the case of hemorrhage due to the blood-iron content. Which pulse sequence would be helpful in identifying hemorrhage?
    ___ a. spin density
    ___ b. gradient echo
    ___ c. T2–weighted images
    ___ d. short tau inversion recovery (STIR)

84. Due to the low development of myelin in pediatric patients, it is very difficult to define gray/white matter structures. Which pulse sequence should be employed?
    ___ a. spin density
    ___ b. gradient echo
    ___ c. proton density
    ___ d. inversion recovery (IR)

85. When scanning a patient's head, the quadrature head coil is most likely used. This configuration indicates that current is transmitted and received through _____ channels or ports.
    ___ a. two
    ___ b. three
    ___ c. four
    ___ d. six

86. Which structures make up the lentiform nucleus?
    ____ a. putamen and globus pallidus
    ____ b. claustrum and caudate nucleus
    ____ c. internal and external capsules
    ____ d. fornix and habenula

87. Which of the following tumors grow slowly and originate from arachnoid tissue? They are routinely hypointense on T1–weighted images.
    ____ a. Chiari malformation
    ____ b. astrocytoma
    ____ c. neurofibroma
    ____ d. meningioma

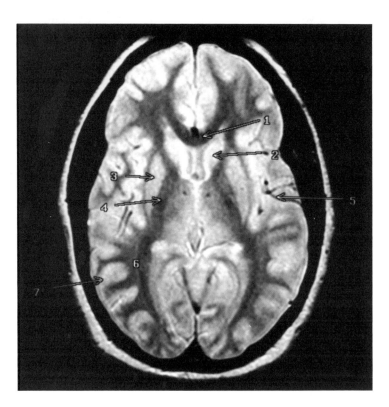

Figure 5

88. Identify the structure marked 1 in Figure 5.

___ a. pineal gland

___ b. anterior cerebral artery

___ c. pituitary

___ d. thalamus

89. Identify structure 2 in Figure 5.

___ a. caudate nucleus

___ b. globus pallidus

___ c. internal capsule

___ d. thalamus

90. Identify 3 in Figure 5.

___ a. caudate nucleus

___ b. globus pallidus

___ c. internal capsule

___ d. external capsule

91. The structure marked 4 in Figure 5 is a _____ structure.

___ a. white matter

___ b. gray matter

___ c. globular

___ d. thalamic

92. Judging from the gray matter appearance in Figure 5, this image was acquired with which pulse sequence?

___ a. T1

___ b. T2

___ c. proton density

___ d. STIR

93. _____ is the vessel denoted by the number 5 on Fig-
    ure 5.
    ____ a. anterior cerebral artery
    ____ b. siphon
    ____ c. middle cerebral artery
    ____ d. none of the above

94. On a soft tissue neck, which structure is in closest proxim-
    ity to the cervical vertebrae?
    ____ a. esophagus
    ____ b. trachea
    ____ c. larynx
    ____ d. pharynx

95. Lymph nodes are frequently _____ and vessels
    are_____ on T1–weighted images of the neck.
    ____ a. gray/bright
    ____ b. dark/bright
    ____ c. isointense/dark
    ____ d. isointense/bright

96. Which of the following is most superior in orientation of
    the pharynx?
    ____ a. cerebropharynx
    ____ b. oropharynx
    ____ c. nasopharynx
    ____ d. laryngopharynx

97. _____ images best demonstrate disk degeneration or
    dehydration.
    ____ a. axial T1
    ____ b. sagittal T1
    ____ c. sagittal T2
    ____ d. none of the above

98. The _____ plane best demonstrates spinal stenosis.
    ____ a. sagittal
    ____ b. axial
    ____ c. coronal
    ____ d. oblique

99. If a patient has had previous lumbar surgery, the _____ sequence should be avoided because susceptibility artifacts are more pronounced in this sequence.
    ____ a. spin echo
    ____ b. gradient echo
    ____ c. fast spin echo
    ____ d. none of the above

100. _____ is the spinal region that is least affected by CSF pulsation.
    ____ a. cervical
    ____ b. thoracic
    ____ c. lumbar
    ____ d. none of the above are affected

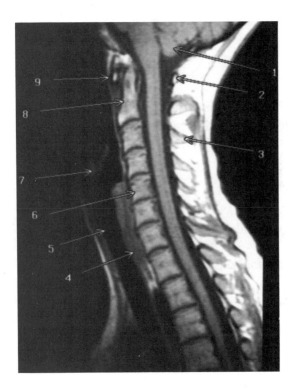

Figure 6

101. Identify structure 1 in Figure 6.
    ____ a. cerebellar tonsil
    ____ b. clivus
    ____ c. cerebral tonsil
    ____ d. pontine tonsil

102. Identify structure 2 in Figure 6.
    ____ a. posterior lymph node
    ____ b. cervical displaced fragment
    ____ c. posterior arch of C1
    ____ d. blood vessel

103. Identify structure 3 in Figure 6.
    ____ a. transverse process
    ____ b. spinous process
    ____ c. pedicle
    ____ d. lamina

104. Identify structure 4 in Figure 6.
    ____ a. esophagus
    ____ b. larynx
    ____ c. pharynx
    ____ d. none of the above

105. Identify structure 7 in Figure 6.
    ____ a. epiglottis
    ____ b. trachea
    ____ c. thyroid
    ____ d. voice box

106. The _____ is the caudal end of the spinal cord.
    ____ a. cauda equina
    ____ b. conus medullaris
    ____ c. filum terminale
    ____ d. all of the above

107. The inferior portion of the spinal cord ends at the _____ level.
    ____ a. T10-T11
    ____ b. T12-L1
    ____ c. L1-L2
    ____ d. sacral

108. The individual nerve roots that leave the caudal portion of the spinal cord progress downward and are called the _____ or the "horse's tail".
    ___ a. filum terminale
    ___ b. cauda equina
    ___ c. uncinate processes
    ___ d. none of the above

109. A condition called _____ is generally found in children in which the cord is pulled lower than its natural level. This may cause tension and difficulty walking.
    ___ a. tethered cord
    ___ b. ruptured cord
    ___ c. strangulated cord
    ___ d. extended cord

110. The CSF in the spinal canal is generally _____ on T1 and _____ on T2.
    ___ a. dark/bright
    ___ b. isointense/isointense
    ___ c. bright/dark
    ___ d. isointense/bright

111. If a patient had a history of galactorrhea, which portion of the brain would you likely image?
    ___ a. pineal gland
    ___ b. cervicocranial junction
    ___ c. pituitary gland
    ___ d. thalamus

112. The appearance of the vertebral body will _____ following fracture or replacement of the bone marrow by infection or neoplasm on T1–weighted images.
    ___ a. have higher signal intensity
    ___ b. have less signal intensity
    ___ c. have a signal that is unaffected
    ___ d. have more vascularity

113. Which plane would best display both the dorsal and ventral nerve roots?

____ a. axial

____ b. sagittal

____ c. coronal

____ d. none of the above

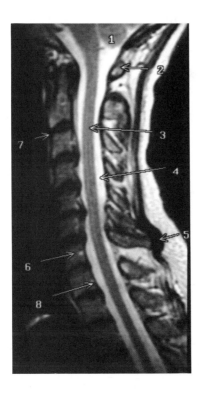

Figure 7

114. Identify structure 4 in Figure 7.

____ a. spinal cord

____ b. CSF

____ c. cauda equina

____ d. anterior longitudinal ligament

115. Identify structure 7 in Figure 7.

      ___ a. posterior longitudinal ligament
      ___ b. anterior longitudinal ligament
      ___ c. transverse longitudinal ligament
      ___ d. spinous ligament

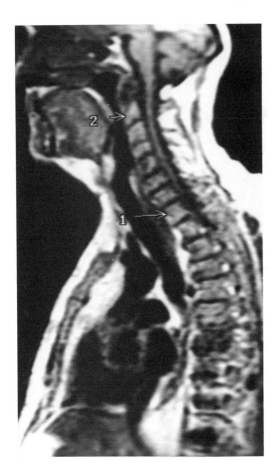

Figure 8

116. Identify structure 1 in Figure 8.

      ___ a. C6
      ___ b. C7
      ___ c. T1
      ___ d. none of the above

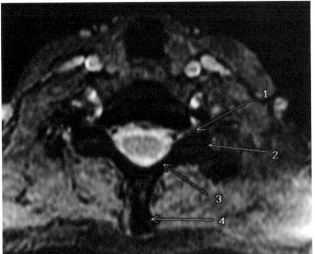

Figure 9

117. Identify number 1 in Figure 9.

   ___ a. lamina

   ___ b. nerve root

   ___ c. pedicle

   ___ d. blood vessel

118. Identify structure 2 in Figure 9.

   ___ a. spinous process

   ___ b. transverse process

   ___ c. vertebral body

   ___ d. lamina

119. Identify structure 3 in Figure 9.

   ___ a. pedicle

   ___ b. lamina

   ___ c. transverse process

   ___ d. spinous process

120. Identify structure 4 in Figure 9.

    ____ a. transverse process

    ____ b. lamina

    ____ c. vertebral body

    ____ d. spinous process

121. Which of the following does not immediately enhance after the injection of contrast?

    ____ a. scar tissue

    ____ b. necrosed tissue

    ____ c. epidural fat

    ____ d. healthy disc

122. A healthy nucleus pulposus generally has a high water content, therefore, you would expect to see a _____ appearance on T2–weighted images.

    ____ a. gray

    ____ b. dark

    ____ c. bright

    ____ d. isointense

123. The _____ is the soft, gelatinous portion of the intervertebral disc.

    ____ a. cauda equina

    ____ b. nucleus pulposus

    ____ c. annulus fibrosus

    ____ d. nucleus fibrosus

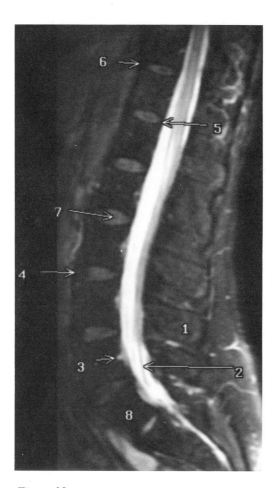

Figure 10

124. Identify figure 2 in Figure 10.

    ____ a. conus medullaris

    ____ b. cauda equina

    ____ c. vertebral body

    ____ d. caudal medullus

125. Identify figure 5 in Figure 10.

    ____ a. transverse longitudinal ligament

    ____ b. anterior longitudinal ligament

    ____ c. posterior longitudinal ligament

    ____ d. filum terminale

126. Identify figure 4 in Figure 10.
    ___ a. vertebral body
    ___ b. nucleus pulposus
    ___ c. annulous fibrosus
    ___ d. annulus pulposus

127. Identify 3 in Figure 10.
    ___ a. venous plexus
    ___ b. ligamentum flavum
    ___ c. anterior facet
    ___ d. annulus fibrosus

128. _____ is the level of the brachial plexus.
    ___ a. C1-T1
    ___ b. C4-T2
    ___ c. C7-T4
    ___ d. T1-T8

129. The nerve roots located in the _____ area are known as the lumbar plexus.
    ___ a. T2-L4
    ___ b. L2-S2
    ___ c. L4-L5
    ___ d. L5-S1

130. Since there is a lack of mobile protons in the lung area, lung tissue is typically _____ on T1– and T2–weighted images.
    ___ a. black
    ___ b. isointense
    ___ c. bright
    ___ d. gray

131. The _____ is the most anterior chamber of the heart seen on cross section.
    ___ a. right ventricle
    ___ b. left ventricle
    ___ c. right atrium
    ___ d. left atrium

132. The _____ is the most posterior chamber of the heart.
    ___ a. left atrium
    ___ b. right atrium
    ___ c. left ventricle
    ___ d. right ventricle

133. The _____ is most readily identified by its thick muscular appearance on axial views of the heart.
    ___ a. left atruim
    ___ b. right atrium
    ___ c. left ventricle
    ___ d. right ventricle

134. Typically, the heart is imaged during _____.
    ___ a. diastole
    ___ b. systole
    ___ c. QRS complex
    ___ d. tamponade

135. The _____ is the level at which the trachea bifurcates into the right and left bronchi.
    ___ a. mediastinum
    ___ b. brachiocephalic juncture
    ___ c. carina
    ___ d. brachiopulmonary juncture

136. The _____ is the only artery that normally carries de-oxygenated blood.

     ____ a. pulmonary artery

     ____ b. renal artery

     ____ c. thoracic aorta

     ____ d. splenic artery

137. The _____ coil is typically used to visualize the thorax.

     ____ a. surface

     ____ b. quadrature T/L

     ____ c. body

     ____ d. extremity

138. Which of the following may be helpful when scanning the thorax?

     ____ a. respiratory gating

     ____ b. cardiac gating

     ____ c. peripheral gating

     ____ d. all of the above

139. It is important to trigger the gating off of the _____.

     ____ a. P wave

     ____ b. R wave

     ____ c. T wave

     ____ d. QRS complex

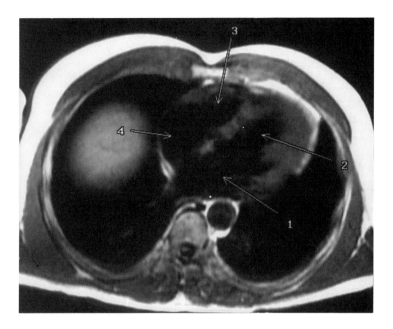

Figure 11

140. Identify structure 2 in Figure 11.
    ___ a. right ventricle
    ___ b. left ventricle
    ___ c. right atrium
    ___ d. left atrium

141. Identify structure 4 in Figure 11.
    ___ a. right ventricle
    ___ b. left ventricle
    ___ c. left atrium
    ___ d. right atrium

142. Identify structure 3 in Figure 11.
    ___ a. right atrium
    ___ b. right ventricle
    ___ c. left atrium
    ___ d. left ventricle

143. The _____ is the largest organ in the abdomen.

  ___ a. stomach

  ___ b. liver

  ___ c. spleen

  ___ d. pancreas

144. Fat, the pancreas, and the spleen are all _____ on T2–weighted images.

  ___ a. hyperintense

  ___ b. gray

  ___ c. black

  ___ d. none of the above

145. Because of its orientation in the abdomen, the _____ plane, displays the pancreas best.

  ___ a. axial

  ___ b. sagittal

  ___ c. coronal

  ___ d. oblique

146. The _____ is a small vein that helps drain the thoracic wall and posterior abdominal wall.

  ___ a. vena cava

  ___ b. azygos vein

  ___ c. pulmonary vein

  ___ d. jugular vein

147. In the abdomen, the protons in water and fat resonate at different frequencies, causing a/an _____ artifact.

  ___ a. chemical shift

  ___ b. susceptibility

  ___ c. aliasing

  ___ d. Gibbs

148. The pancreas, duodenum, lymph nodes, adrenal glands, and the kidneys are all located in the _____ cavity.
    ___ a. thoracic
    ___ b. abdominal
    ___ c. pelvic
    ___ d. retroperitoneal

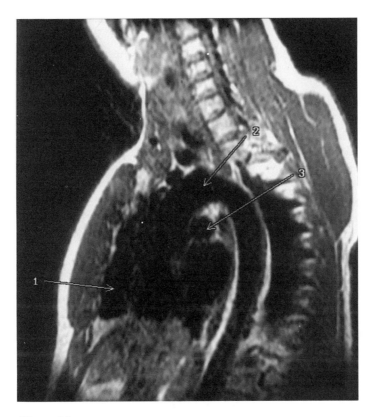

Figure 12

149. Identify arrow 1 in Figure 12.
    ___ a. Right ventricle
    ___ b. Right atrium
    ___ c. Left ventricle
    ___ d. Left atrium

150. Which of the following are important to remember when scanning the breast?

_____ a. acquire high resolution in all three imaging planes

_____ b. employ fat suppression techniques to differentiate fat from tumor

_____ c. all of the breast tissue should be included, especially the tissue nearest the sternum

_____ d. all of the above

151. Which of the following techniques are employed post contrast when visualizing the breast.

_____ a. T2–weighted images

_____ b. T1–weighted images

_____ c. T1–weighted images with fat saturation

_____ d. Inversion recovery (IR) images

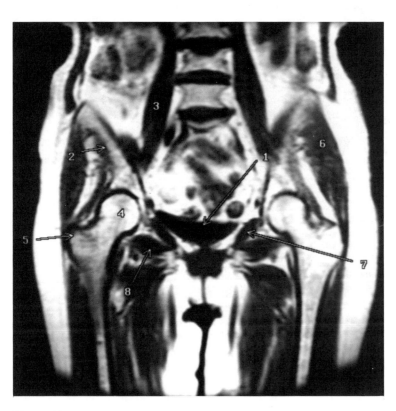

Figure 13

152. Identify structure 3 in Figure 13.
    ___ a. psoas muscle
    ___ b. gluteal muscle
    ___ c. obturator muscle
    ___ d. iliac muscle

153. Identify structure 5 in Figure 13.
    ___ a. humeral head
    ___ b. femoral head
    ___ c. greater trochanter
    ___ d. lesser trochanter

154. Identify structure 7 in Figure 13.
    ___ a. psoas muscle
    ___ b. gluteal muscle
    ___ c. obturator externus
    ___ d. obturator internus

155. Identify structure 2 in Figure 13.
    ___ a. ilium
    ___ b. acetabulum
    ___ c. pubic symphysis
    ___ d. sacrum

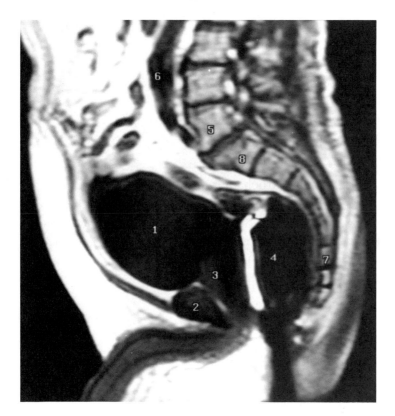

Figure 14

156. Identify structure 1 in Figure 14 .

    ____ a. bowel

    ____ b. uterus

    ____ c. placenta

    ____ d. bladder

157. Identify structure 2 in Figure 14.

    ____ a. scrotum

    ____ b. seminal vesicles

    ____ c. prostate

    ____ d. pubic symphysis

158. Identify structure 3 in Figure 14.

    ____ a. prostate

    ____ b. prostrate

    ____ c. bladder

    ____ d. cervix

159. Identify structure 4 in Figure 14.

    ____ a. endorectal coil

    ____ b. rectum

    ____ c. bowel

    ____ d. prostate

160. Identify structure 6 in Figure 14.

    ____ a. bowel

    ____ b. thoracic aorta

    ____ c. psoas muscle

    ____ d. rectum

161. Which coil should be used to display the pelvis on an adult ?

    ____ a. quadrature T/L coil

    ____ b. body coil

    ____ c. surface coil

    ____ d. endorectal coil

162. Which coil is most useful when scanning the prostate?

    ____ a. quadrature T/L coil

    ____ b. body coil

    ____ c. surface coil

    ____ d. endorectal coil

163. Which pulse sequence would best display a bone bruise in the knee area?

    ____ a. T1 spin density

    ____ b. T2 spin density

    ____ c. gradient-recalled acquisition

    ____ d. IR

164. State conditions which may be contraindications for the use of gadolinium.

_____ a. sickle cell anemia

_____ b. hemolytic anemia

_____ c. renal failure

_____ d. none known

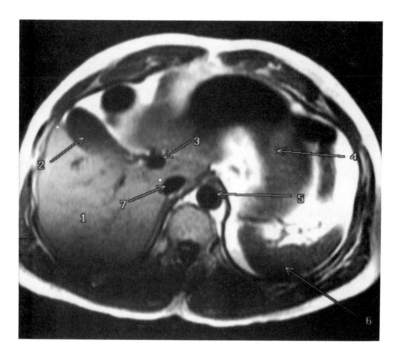

Figure 15

165. Identify structure 1 in Figure 15.

_____ a. liver

_____ b. stomach

_____ c. lung

_____ d. bowel

166. Identify structure 2 in Figure 15.

_____ a. spleen

_____ b. gallbladder

_____ c. adrenal

_____ d. bowel

167. Identify structure 3 in Figure 15.

    ____ a. aorta

    ____ b. vena cava

    ____ c. hepatic vein

    ____ d. portal vein

168. Identify structure 4 in Figure 15.

    ____ a. bowel

    ____ b. spleen

    ____ c. stomach

    ____ d. pancreas

169. Identify structure 6 in Figure 15.

    ____ a. spleen

    ____ b. stomach

    ____ c. pancreas

    ____ d. liver

170. Identify structure 7 in Figure 15.

    ____ a. aorta

    ____ b. inferior vena cava

    ____ c. portal vein

    ____ d. renal vein

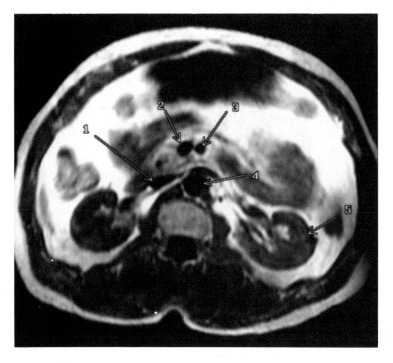

Figure 16

171. Identify structure 5 in Figure 16.

_____ a. renal cortex

_____ b. renal medulla

_____ c. adrenal gland

_____ d. spleen

172. Identify structure 4 in Figure 16.

_____ a. aorta

_____ b. vena cava

_____ c. azygos vein

_____ d. coronary artery

173. Identify structure 3 in Figure 16.

_____ a. portal vein

_____ b. hepatic vein

_____ c. superior mesenteric artery

_____ d. superior mesenteric vein

174. _____ is the effective dosage of gadolinium.
    ___ a. 0.2 mL/kg
    ___ b. 0.1 mM/kg
    ___ c. 0.1 mL/lb
    ___ d. all of the above

175. Approximately 80% of gadolinium is excreted by the kidneys in _____ hours.
    ___ a. 2
    ___ b. 3
    ___ c. 6
    ___ d. 8

176. Which coil is used to visualize the shoulder?
    ___ a. extremity coil
    ___ b. body coil
    ___ c. bird cage
    ___ d. surface coil

177. Which coil is typically used to image the TMJ?
    ___ a. head coil
    ___ b. body coil
    ___ c. extremity coil
    ___ d. 3" surface coil

178. _____ is used to display the range of motion on a temporomandibular joint (TMJ).
    ___ a. cardiac device
    ___ b. kinematic device
    ___ c. maximum intensity pixel device
    ___ d. none of the above

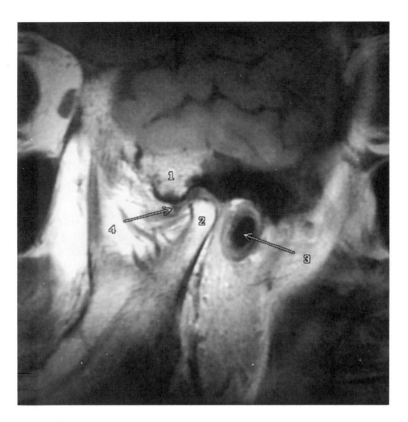

Figure 17

179. Identify structure labeled 3 in Figure 17.

___ a. carotid artery

___ b. Meckel's cave

___ c. external meatus

___ d. parotid gland

180. Identify structure labeled 4 in Figure 17.

___ a. meniscus

___ b. labrum

___ c. condular cartilage

___ d. capsular ligament

181. When scanning the brain, the landmark should be at the
    _____ level.

    ___ a. orbital
    ___ b. canthomeatal
    ___ c. external meatal
    ___ d. nasion

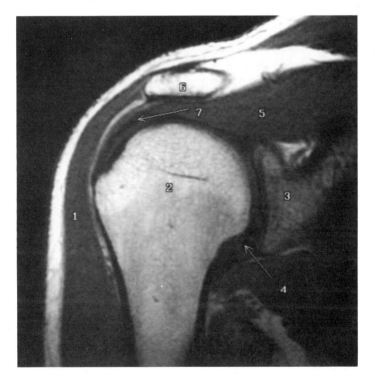

Figure 18

182. Identify structure 1 in Figure 18.

    ___ a. deltoid muscle
    ___ b. trapezius muscle
    ___ c. supraspinatus muscle
    ___ d. subscapularis muscle

183. Identify structure 2 in Figure 18.
    ____ a. greater trochanter
    ____ b. femoral head
    ____ c. lesser trochanter
    ____ d. humeral head

184. Identify structure 3 in Figure 18.
    ____ a. clavicle
    ____ b. acromion
    ____ c. glenoid fossa
    ____ d. deltoid fossa

185. Identify structure 4 in Figure 18.
    ____ a. labrum
    ____ b. coracoid cartilage
    ____ c. glenoid fossa
    ____ d. supraspinatus tendon

186. Identify structure 5 in Figure 18.
    ____ a. supraspinatus tendon
    ____ b. supraspinatus muscle
    ____ c. infraspinatus muscle
    ____ d. deltoid muscle

187. Identify structure 6 in Figure 18.
    ____ a. acromion
    ____ b. glenoid fossa
    ____ c. coracoid process
    ____ d. labrum

188. Figure 18 is in the _____ projection.
    ____ a. axial
    ____ b. off-axis coronal
    ____ c. off-axis sagittal
    ____ d. true sagittal

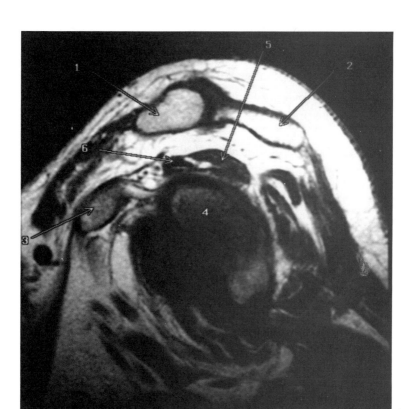

Figure 19

189. Figure 19 is in the _____ position.

_____ a. axial

_____ b. off-axis coronal

_____ c. off-axis sagittal

_____ d. true coronal

190. Identify structure 1 in Figure 19.

_____ a. glenoid fossa

_____ b. acromion

_____ c. subscapularis

_____ d. clavicle

191. Which of the following make up the rotator cuff?

    ____ a. deltoid, pectoralis major, latissimus dorsi

    ____ b. deltoid, biceps, subscapularis

    ____ c. supraspinatus, infraspinatus, teres minor,
         subscapularis

    ____ d. supraspinatus, infraspinatus, subscapularis

192. Which coil is generally used to display the knee?

    ____ a. surface coil

    ____ b. extremity coil

    ____ c. quadrature head coil

    ____ d. body coil

193. _____ is the position which best demonstrates the
     anterior cruciate ligament.

    ____ a. neutral position

    ____ b. 5-10° internal rotation

    ____ c. 15° external rotation

    ____ d. 45° external rotation

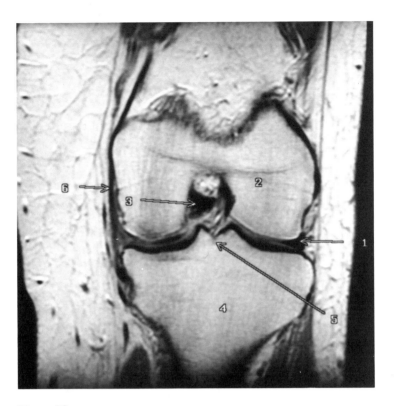

Figure 20

194. The anatomy in Figure 20 is in the _____ position.

    ____ a. axial

    ____ b. sagittal

    ____ c. coronal

    ____ d. off axis sagittal

195. Identify structure 3 in Figure 20.

    ____ a. medial collateral ligament

    ____ b. anterior cruciate ligament

    ____ c. posterior cruciate ligament

    ____ d. popliteal artery

196. Identify structure 4 in Figure 20.

_____ a. femur

_____ b. humerus

_____ c. tibia

_____ d. fibula

197. The fibula is on the same side as structure 1 in Figure 20. Identify this structure.

_____ a. lateral meniscus

_____ b. medial meniscus

_____ c. lateral collateral ligament

_____ d. medial collateral ligament

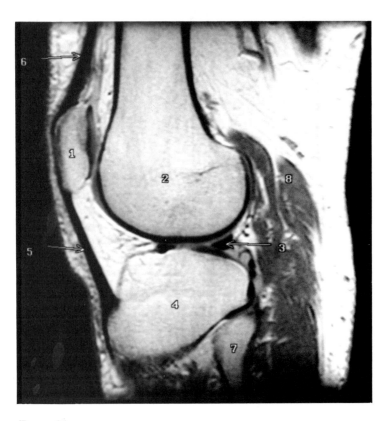

Figure 21

198. Identify structure 6 in Figure 21.
    ___ a. patellar ligament
    ___ b. quadriceps tendon
    ___ c. anterior cruciate ligament
    ___ d. popliteal tendon

199. Identify structure 1 in Figure 21.
    ___ a. patella
    ___ b. condyle
    ___ c. tibia
    ___ d. fibula

200. Identify structure 4 in Figure 21.
    ___ a. humeru
    ___ b. fibula
    ___ c. tibia
    ___ d. femur

201. Identify structure 7 in Figure 21.
    ___ a. humerus
    ___ b. fibula
    ___ c. tibia
    ___ d. femur

202. Identify structure 5 in Figure 21.
    ___ a. patellar tendon
    ___ b. quadriceps tendon
    ___ c. popliteal tendon
    ___ d. femoral tendon

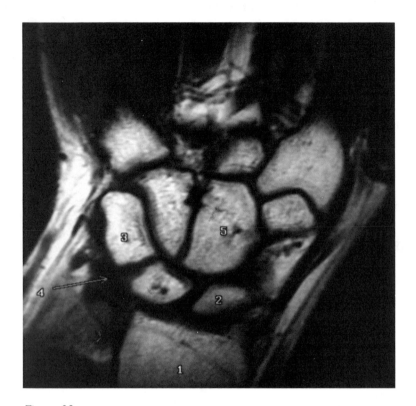

Figure 22

203. Identify structure 1 in Figure 22.

___ a. ulna

___ b. radius

___ c. 2nd metacarpal

___ d. olecranon

204. Identify structure 4 in Figure 22.

___ a. triquetrum

___ b. scaphoid

___ c. triangular fibrocartilage

___ d. ulnar fibrocartilage

205. Imaging in the _____ plane best demonstrates compression within the carpal tunnel.

    ___ a. axial

    ___ b. coronal

    ___ c. sagittal

    ___ d. off-axis sagittal

206. _____ is a condition in which there has been a cessation of blood to a bony part, causing a portion of the bone to die.

    ___ a. avascular necrosis (AVN)

    ___ b. arteriovenous malformation (AVM)

    ___ c. hematoma

    ___ d. none of the above

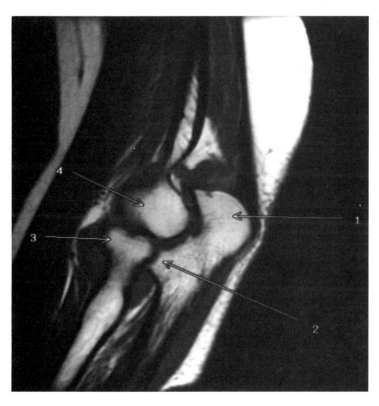

Figure 23

207. Identify structure 1 in Figure 23.
    ____ a. coronoid process
    ____ b. capitullum
    ____ c. capitellum
    ____ d. olecranon

208. Identify structure 3 in Figure 23.
    ____ a. radial head
    ____ b. capitellum
    ____ c. olecranon
    ____ d. ulnar head

209. Identify structure 2 in Figure 23.
    ____ a. capitellum
    ____ b. radial head
    ____ c. olecranon
    ____ d. coronoid

210. Identify structure 4 in Figure 23.
    ____ a. olecranon
    ____ b. trochlea
    ____ c. capitellum
    ____ d. epicondyle

Pulse Sequences

211. What is the time interval between the 90° RF pulse and a subsequent 90° RF pulse applied to the same slice?
    ____ a. TD
    ____ b. TI
    ____ c. TE
    ____ d. TR

212. What is the time interval between the 90° RF pulse and the first echo?
    ____ a. TR
    ____ b. TE
    ____ c. TD
    ____ d. TI

213. What parameters are used to create spin echo (SE) T2-weighted images?
    ____ a. short TE and short TR
    ____ b. short TE and long TR
    ____ c. long TE and long TR
    ____ d. long TE and short TR

214. What mechanism rephases the dephasing hydrogen nuclei in a SE sequence?
    ____ a. 180° RF pulse
    ____ b. 90° RF pulse
    ____ c. the free induction decay signal (FID)
    ____ d. gradient reversal after the 90° RF pulse

215. What function does the initial 180° RF pulse have in an IR pulse sequence?
    ____ a. dephases the net magnetization vector
    ____ b. flips the net magnetization into the negative longitudinal plane for greater T1 relaxation range
    ____ c. is followed by the collection of the echo
    ____ d. suppresses the signal from fat

216. Gradient recalled echo (GRE) pulse sequences are accomplished using the following events:
    ____ a. 90° RF, 180° RF, 180° RF pulses
    ____ b. 180° RF pulse, gradient reversal
    ____ c. 90° RF pulse, gradient reversal
    ____ d. less than 90° RF pulse, gradient reversal

217. What do spin density images measure?
    ____ a. magnetic susceptibility
    ____ b. a subset of all protons in fat and water molecules
    ____ c. specific absorption rate
    ____ d. magnetic field strength

218. Which RF pulse series produces several true T2-weighted SE images with each TR?
    ____ a. a 90° RF pulse, a series of 180° RF pulses and the collection of echoes
    ____ b. a series of 90° RF pulses followed by the collection of an echo
    ____ c. a series of 180° RF pulses followed by the collection of echoes
    ____ d. a 23° RF pulse followed by the collection of echoes

219. What are the additional RF pulses called that are used to saturate out hydrogen nuclei prior to excitation?
    ____ a. oversaturation
    ____ b. presaturation
    ____ c. flow compensation
    ____ d. magnetic moment

220. What is the term for the time from the excitation pulse to the refocusing pulse and from the refocusing pulse to the echo?
    ____ a. time delay
    ____ b. dead time
    ____ c. tau time
    ____ d. interpulse time

221. In an SE, what is the term for the time between the 90°
     RF pulse and the 180° RF pulse?
     1. TE
     2. tau
     3. TE/2

     ____ a. 1 only
     ____ b. 2 only
     ____ c. 2 and 3 only
     ____ d. 1, 2, and 3

222. What is the image quality result on SE images if the TE
     is lengthened?
     ____ a. increases the contrast based on the T2 of the tis-
             sues
     ____ b. reduces the contrast based on the T2 of the tis-
             sues
     ____ c. reduces the contrast based on the T1 of the tis-
             sues
     ____ d. increases the contrast based on the T1 of the tis-
             sues

223. In a GRE sequence, if the flip angle is lowered while
     holding the TR constant, which of the following would
     be reduced?
     ____ a. chemical shift artifact
     ____ b. magnetic susceptibility
     ____ c. saturation
     ____ d. scan time

224. Which of these pulse sequences is the most "flow sensi-
     tive"?
     ____ a. SE
     ____ b. GRE
     ____ c. IR
     ____ d. Short TI Inversion Recovery (STIR)

225. What term describes the signal that follows the application of the initial 90° RF pulse?

_____ a. spin echo

_____ b. gradient echo

_____ c. FID

_____ d. Hahn echo

226. Due to the decreased efficiency in refocusing spins, this pulse sequence is extremely sensitive to magnetic field homogeneity:

_____ a. SE

_____ b. GRE

_____ c. IR

_____ d. Three Dimensional Fourier Transform (3DFT) SE

227. What will be the effect of shortening the TE time?

1. increases signal-to-noise ratio (SNR)
2. increases the spin density contrast weighting
3. reduces contrast based on T2 relaxation times

_____ a. 1 only

_____ b. 3 only

_____ c. 2 and 3 only

_____ d. 1, 2, and 3

228. Which of these statements is true regarding spoiled GRE sequences?

1. spoils the transverse signal
2. increases T2* dependence
3. only longitudinal signals contribute to next RF pulse

_____ a. 1 only

_____ b. 3 only

_____ c. 1 and 2 only

_____ d. 1 and 3 only

229. A long TR msec (3000 msec or greater) and a short TE (shorter than 40 msec) would acquire an image that would produce which type of image contrast?
    ___ a. T1-weighted
    ___ b. T2-weighted
    ___ c. T2*-weighted
    ___ d. proton density-weighted (PD-weighted)

230. What is the correct formula for determining the total scan time, in minutes, for a 3DFT image?
    ___ a. TR (sec) x TE x Number of excitations (NEX) x Number of phase encoding steps (Npe)
    ___ b. TR (sec) x TE x Npe x NEX x Number of slices (Nslices)/60,000 (msec)
    ___ c. TR (msec) x Npe x NEX/60 (sec)
    ___ d. TR (sec) x Npe x NEX x Nslices/60 (sec)

231. What type of pulse sequence begins with a 90° RF pulse and is immediately followed by the collection of the echo?
    ___ a. spin echo
    ___ b. inversion recovery
    ___ c. short TI inversion recovery
    ___ d. partial saturation

232. What is a way to reduce the scan time without directly affecting image contrast?
    ___ a. reduce the TR
    ___ b. reduce the Npe
    ___ c. use a gradient reversal
    ___ d. reduce the TE

233. The peak signal strength of a spin echo is less than the initial strength of the FID because of _____.
    ___ a. magnetic susceptibility
    ___ b. T1 relaxation
    ___ c. T2 relaxation
    ___ d. proton concentration

234. Which of these statements are true regarding rephased GRE pulse sequences?
    1. rephased GRE sequences preserve transverse signal
    2. both longitudinal and transverse signals contribute to the next RF pulse
    3. rephased GRE sequences increase T1 dependence

    ____ a. 1 only
    ____ b. 2 only
    ____ c. 1 and 2 only
    ____ d. 1 and 3 only

235. Place the following SE pulse sequence events in the correct order.
    1. signal measurement
    2. 180° RF pulse
    3. 90° RF pulse

    ____ a. 1, 2, 3
    ____ b. 2, 1, 3
    ____ c. 3, 2, 1
    ____ d. 1, 3, 2

236. What is the term for an echo formed by the application of two successive 90° RF pulses?
    ____ a. partial saturation echo
    ____ b. Hahn echo
    ____ c. spin echo
    ____ d. gradient recalled echo

237. Changing the TR will directly affect which of the following?
    ____ a. slice thickness
    ____ b. orientation of the image plane
    ____ c. acquisition time
    ____ d. field of view

238. Which of these statements is not true regarding steady state?

    ____ a. The TR must be shorter than the T1 and T2 of the tissues.

    ____ b. The TR must equal the tau of the spin echo.

    ____ c. During the acquisition, the flip angle and the TR maintain the steady state.

    ____ d. all of the above are true statements

239. What is the term for the distance traveled between the positive and negative lobe of the velocity-encoding gradient?

    ____ a. velocity

    ____ b. turbulence

    ____ c. gradient moment nulling

    ____ d. laminar flow

240. Regarding flow, which of these causes a decrease in signal intensity?

    1. high-flow void
    2. turbulence
    3. diastolic pseudogating

    ____ a. 1 only

    ____ b. 1 and 2 only

    ____ c. 2 only

    ____ d. 1, 2, and 3

241. Using flip angles of 10° or less in a GRE pulse sequence will result in what effect on the image?

    ____ a. less T2*-weighting

    ____ b. less SNR

    ____ c. longer relaxation times

    ____ d. more T1-weighting

242. Coherent, incoherent, and steady state free precession (SSFP) pulse sequences can be differentiated according

to whether or not they use the FID or spin echo signals. Which statement is correct?

1. Coherent pulse sequences use a gradient reversal to rephase both the FID and the dephasing portion of the spin echo.

2. Incoherent pulse sequences use a gradient reversal to rephase both the FID and rephasing portion of the spin echo.

3. SSFP uses an RF pulse to initiate the rephasing process and a rewinder to move the spin echo to occur before the RF pulse.

_____ a. 2 only

_____ b. 3 only

_____ c. 2 and 3 only

_____ d. 1 and 3 only

243. Which of the following pulse sequences allow tissues to relax over twice the dynamic range possible with SE pulse sequence?

_____ a. 45° GRE

_____ b. 3DFT

_____ c. EPI

_____ d. IR

244. If the TR is reduced, how is the image quality affected?

1. SNR decreases.

2. T2 contrast increases.

3. Spin density weighting is increased.

_____ a. 1 only

_____ b. 3 only

_____ c. 1 and 2 only

_____ d. 1 and 3 only

245. In a CSE pulse sequence, a 90° RF pulse is followed by a 180° RF pulse. How much more power does it take to deliver a 180° RF pulse compared with the 90° RF pulse?

    ____ a. twice

    ____ b. half

    ____ c. quadruple

    ____ d. eight times

246. In an IR pulse sequence, what is the term for the time between the initial 180° and the 90° RF pulse?

    ____ a. TE

    ____ b. TR

    ____ c. TI

    ____ d. T1

Data Manipulation

247. SNR is proportional to which of the following?

    1. $\sqrt{NEX}$

    2. $\dfrac{1}{\sqrt{(received\ bandwidth)}}$

    3. $\dfrac{1}{(number\ of\ phase\ encodings)}$

    ____ a. 1 only

    ____ b. 1 and 3 only

    ____ c. 1 and 2 only

    ____ d. 1, 2, and 3 only

248. In a CSE pulse sequence, the 180° RF pulse flips the net magnetization 180 degrees into the opposite direction. In a GRE pulse sequence, what effect does a gradient reversal have on net magnetization?

    ____ a. spins that have slowed down speed up, and vice versa, allowing remaining net magnetization to rephase

    ____ b. the spins flip 180° in the opposite direction

    ____ c. the spins rephase immediately and return their signal faster

    ____ d. it has no effect on CSE pulse sequences

249. For a GRE pulse sequence with a 45° flip angle, what is the total power deposited per TR compared with a CSE pulse sequence?

    ____ a. 5%

    ____ b. 12.5%

    ____ c. 25%

    ____ d. 50%

250. What is it called when only half the area of the k-space is filled along the frequency axis?
    ___ a. zero filling
    ___ b. fractional echo
    ___ c. partial acquisition
    ___ d. partial averaging

251. Reducing the receive bandwidth causes what result(s)?
    1. less noise is sampled
    2. SNR increases
    3. minimum TE available increases

    ___ a. 1 only
    ___ b. 1 and 2 only
    ___ c. 2 and 3 only
    ___ d. 1, 2, and 3

252. Why are presaturation pulses useful?
    ___ a. to improve spatial resolution
    ___ b. to reduce flow artifacts
    ___ c. to reduce scan time
    ___ d. to turn flowing blood bright

253. Where in the pulse sequence are presaturation pulses usually placed?
    ___ a. prior to the excitation pulse
    ___ b. after the 180° RF pulse
    ___ c. between the 90° and 180° RF pulse
    ___ d. after the excitation pulse

254. The highest amplitude signal is stored in which area of k-space?
    ___ a. on the outer lines of k-space
    ___ b. on the central lines of k-space
    ___ c. only on the center line of k-space
    ___ d. on the bottom half of k-space

255. The receive bandwidth is related to the slope of which gradient?

___ a. read out
___ b. phase encoding
___ c. slice-selecting
___ d. transmitting

256. What is 10 mT/m, the typical gradient strength, equal to in G/cm?

___ a. .01 G/cm
___ b. .1 G/cm
___ c. 1 G/cm
___ d. 10 G/cm

257. What is the term that describes the finite amount of time required for the gradient to reach its full amplitude after the power is applied?

___ a. gradient slope
___ b. gradient amplitude
___ c. rise time
___ d. amplitude time

258. The presence of random noise means that doubling the NEX increases the SNR by what factor?

1. $\sqrt{2}$
2. 1.41
3. 2

___ a. 1 only
___ b. 2 only
___ c. 3 only
___ d. 1 and 2 only

259. The highest spatial resolution of the image is located where in k-space?
　　 ___ a. on the outer lines of k-space
　　 ___ b. on the central lines of k-space
　　 ___ c. only on the center line of k-space
　　 ___ d. on the top half of k-space

260. What is the term for the number of times data is collected with the same phase encoding gradient amplitude slope?
　　 ___ a. TR
　　 ___ b. excitation
　　 ___ c. phase encode step
　　 ___ d. NEX or number of averages

261. How does a reduced receiver bandwidth affect the length of time the frequency encoding gradient is on?
　　 ___ a. increases it
　　 ___ b. decreases it
　　 ___ c. has no effect on it
　　 ___ d. cannot change

262. When sinc-shaped RF pulses are Fourier transformed, what slice and pulse profile results would be expected?
　　 1. slice profile is square in shape
　　 2. pulse profiles permit nearly contiguous slices
　　 3. slice profile is gaussian in shape

　　 ___ a. 1 only
　　 ___ b. 1 and 2 only
　　 ___ c. 2 and 3 only
　　 ___ d. 3 only

263. SNR is proportional to:

____ a. $\frac{pixel\ area}{FOV^2}$, $\sqrt{NEX}$, and $\frac{1}{(receive\ bandwidth)}$

____ b. TR, proton density, and $\frac{1}{(\#\ of\ frequency\ encodings)}$

____ c. $\frac{1}{(number\ of\ frequency\ encodings)}$, slice thickness, and flip angle

____ d. TE, $\frac{1}{\sqrt{NEX}}$, and slice thickness

264. In a 3D acquisition, how are the slices produced?

____ a. by applying a slice-select gradient for as many slices as requested

____ b. by applying multiple 180° pulses along the slice-selection (z) direction

____ c. by sampling multiple lines of k-space per pulse sequence

____ d. using very accurate RF pulses

265. In Time of Flight (TOF) magnetic resonance angiography, a 2D or 3D imaging volume is pulsed rapidly so that full recovery of longitudinal magnetization is not possible between excitations and causes a phenomenon called?

___ a. masking
___ b. saturation
___ c. maximum intensity
___ d. steady state

266. Which of the conditions below would we expect with 3D TOF?

___ a. background objects with extremely short T1 characteristics may fail to be fully saturated
___ b. acquisition times are short enough for breath-hold abdominal imaging
___ c. longer TE times are required due to the acquisition process
___ d. the sequence is not limited by FOV

267. Which of these statements is/are true regarding vascular imaging?

1. The longer the TE the greater the likelihood that vascular signal will be lost in the area of a stenosis or after a rapid bend.
2. Larger voxels mean a larger quantity of spins, increasing the likelihood that spins will randomly cancel.
3. Due to the imperfect rectangular slice profile, all 3D acquisitions have one or a few poor images at the edge of the slab.

___ a. 3 only
___ b. 1 and 3 only
___ c. 2 and 3 only
___ d. 1, 2, and 3

268. Which term below is used to describe a record of a maximum intensity ray as it passes through an angiographic volume?

____ a. rephase/dephase

____ b. maximum intensity projection (MIP)

____ c. subtraction techniques

____ d. none of the above

269. What do MRA images depict?

____ a. an anatomical map of the vessel lumen

____ b. a physiologic record of blood flow

____ c. an angiographic visualization of stationary tissues

____ d. all of the above

270. What is the normal range of human peak systolic blood flow velocities?

____ a. 20-175 cm/sec

____ b. 60-300 cm/sec

____ c. 90-460 cm/sec

____ d. 150-500 cm/sec

271. Which vessel has the highest peak systolic blood flow?

____ a. carotid arteries

____ b. middle and anterior cerebral arteries

____ c. ascending aorta

____ d. distal aorta

272. What is predictable distribution of flow velocities in layers that parallel the vessel wall called?

____ a. turbulent flow

____ b. laminar flow

____ c. vortex flow

____ d. vascular flow

273. Localized swirling or stagnant blood flow that has separated from the central streamlines within a vessel is called
_____.

___ a. turbo flow
___ b. plug flow
___ c. laminar flow
___ d. vortex flow

274. What term describes signal variations resulting from the motion of protons flowing into or out of an imaging volume during a given pulse sequence?

___ a. spin-related enhancement
___ b. TOF effects
___ c. saturation
___ d. none of the above

275. Two different flow-related signal changes occur when evenly spaced spin echoes are acquired. This causes loss of signal after odd-numbered echoes and an increased signal on even-numbered echoes. What is this phenomenon called?

___ a. high velocity signal loss
___ b. flow-related enhancement
___ c. even-echo rephasing
___ d. paradoxical enhancement

276. In which portions of the circulatory system is turbulent flow seen?

1. vascular bifurcation
2. aorta
3. distal to areas of stenosis

___ a. 1 only
___ b. 1 and 2 only
___ c. 2 only
___ d. 1, 2, and 3

277. In this process an imaging volume is repeatedly subjected to RF pulses that flip the longitudinal magnetization into the transverse plane, thus decreasing the tissue's signal.
    ____ a. TOF effects
    ____ b. saturation
    ____ c. high-velocity signal loss
    ____ d. none of the above

278. What is the term used when blood velocities exceed a critical threshold and disrupt the laminar flow state?
    ____ a. turbulent flow
    ____ b. plug flow
    ____ c. laminar flow
    ____ d. vortex flow

279. In the imaging process, which physical component causes the induced phase shift to be proportional to position?
    ____ a. static magnetic field
    ____ b. RF
    ____ c. magnetic field gradient
    ____ d. imaging pulse sequence

280. For constant flow in a long, straight vessel with no branching, blood flow is typically which of the following patterns?
    ____ a. pulsatile
    ____ b. laminar
    ____ c. complex
    ____ d. turbulent

281. TOF effects in MR arise from the movement of what?
    ____ a. the net magnetic vector
    ____ b. longitudinal magnetization
    ____ c. transverse magnetization
    ____ d. magnetic field gradient

282. During a single pulse sequence repetition, what causes flow-induced phase shift effects?
    1. the phase of transverse magnetization as blood moves along a gradient
    2. longitudinal magnetization as blood moves along a gradient
    3. blood motion over a distance during a gradient pulse

    ___ a. 1 only
    ___ b. 2 only
    ___ c. 1 and 3 only
    ___ d. 2 and 3 only

283. By increasing the TE from 80 msec to 120 msec on a SE pulse sequence, which of the following is expected?

_____ a. fewer protons experience spin-spin interactions

_____ b. better tissue contrast based on the tissues' T2 characteristics

_____ c. a stronger signal in the MR echo

_____ d. better tissue contrast based on the tissues' T1 characteristics

284. By decreasing the TR from 1000 msec to 500 msec on a SE pulse sequence, which of the following is expected?

_____ a. fewer protons experience spin-spin interactions

_____ b. better tissue contrast based on the tissues' T2 characteristics

_____ c. a stronger signal in the MR echo

_____ d. better tissue contrast based on the tissues' T1 characteristics

285. If six successive 180° RF pulses are applied, following a 90° RF pulse, how many echoes are formed?

_____ a. one

_____ b. three

_____ c. five

_____ d. six

286. If six successive 180° RF pulses are applied, following a 90° RF pulse, which resulting echo will contain the greatest signal?

_____ a. first

_____ b. second

_____ c. third

_____ d. sixth

287. Following dephasing, which of the following RF flip angles maximizes the component of the net magnetization in the transverse plane at the time of the spin echo?

_____ a. 45°

_____ b. 90°

_____ c. 120°

_____ d. 180°

288. Steep gradients are used to produce which of the following results?

1. small FOV
2. thin slices
3. fine matrix

_____ a. 1 only

_____ b. 1 and 2 only

_____ c. 2 and 3 only

_____ d. 1, 2, and 3

289. SNR increases in a 3D-sequence when which other parameter is increased?

_____ a. FOV

_____ b. slab thickness

_____ c. TE

_____ d. a or b

290. Which of the following dephasing mechanisms presents with a void of signal on the high-frequency side and an addition of signal on the low-frequency side of the organ?

_____ a. chemical shift

_____ b. magnetic susceptibility

_____ c. magnetic field inhomogeneities

_____ d. spin-spin interactions

291. Which of the following parameters control the amount of contrast seen in an image due to T2 relaxation?

____ a. TI

____ b. TE

____ c. TR

____ d. TD

292. Which of the following parameters control the amount of contrast seen in an image due to T1 relaxation?

____ a. tau

____ b. TE

____ c. TR

____ d. TD

293. If three 180° RF pulses are applied to generate three echoes, which of the following is/are responsible for the third echo being smaller than the first echo?

____ a. spin-spin interactions

____ b. magnetic susceptibility

____ c. magnetic field inhomogeneities

____ d. all of these

294. Even echo rephasing can only occur if which of the following parameters are used?

____ a. single echoes

____ b. asymmetric echoes

____ c. symmetric echoes

____ d. gradient echoes

295. Presaturation pulses are used to:

1. reduce patient breathing motion
2. reduce flow artifacts
3. increase the FOV

____ a. 1 only

____ b. 2 only

____ c. 1 and 2 only

____ d. 1, 2, and 3

296. Reducing the NEX reduces the scan time and causes what effect on SNR?

____ a. reduction

____ b. increase

____ c. no effect

____ d. doubling

297. Why is SNR proportional to the square root of measurements and not just to the number of measurements?

1. Signal strength itself is proportional to the number of measurements.
2. Noise increases only with the square root of the number of measurements.
3. Image noise covers a wide range of frequencies and is uncorrelated measurement to measurement.

____ a. 1 only

____ b. 3 only

____ c. 1 and 3 only

____ d. 1, 2, and 3

298. If the velocity encoding (VENC) value for phase contrast MRA is set too high, what results would be expected?

1. The range of flows imaged have only a limited number of degrees of phase shift.
2. SNR will not be as high.
3. Vessels with slow flow may be difficult to see.

____ a. 1 only

____ b. 1 and 2

____ c. 2 and 3

____ d. 1, 2, and 3

299. Reducing the FOV by a factor of 2 reduces the voxel volume by what factor?

____ a. $\sqrt{2}$

____ b. 2

____ c. 8

____ d. 4

300. SNR increases as which of the following occur?
    1. receiver bandwidth decreases
    2. receiver bandwidth increases
    3. sampling time increases

    ____ a. 1 only
    ____ b. 2 only
    ____ c. 1 and 3 only
    ____ d. 2 and 3 only

301. Decreasing the receiver bandwidth has what affect on SNR?

    ____ a. decreases it
    ____ b. inverts it
    ____ c. increases it
    ____ d. has no effect on it

302. Pixel area is determined by the size of the FOV and the number of pixels in the FOV and can be calculated by using which of the following equations?

    ____ a. pixel = matrix x FOV
    ____ b. pixel = FOV/matrix
    ____ c. pixel = matrix/FOV
    ____ d. a and b

303. Increasing the TR will have what affect on the image?
    1. increase T2-weighting contrast
    2. decrease T1-weighting contrast
    3. increase SNR

    ____ a. 1 and 3 only
    ____ b. 2 and 3 only
    ____ c. 1, 2, and 3
    ____ d. none of the above

304. How will tissues with loosely bound hydrogen protons appear on T2-weighted images?

___ a. bright
___ b. dark
___ c. gray
___ d. none of the above

305. T1 relaxation is manipulated by which of the following parameters?

1. TR
2. TE
3. flip angle

___ a. 1 only
___ b. 1 and 2 only
___ c. 1 and 3 only
___ d. 1, 2, and 3

306. T2 relaxation depends on which of the following imaging parameters?

1. TR
2. TE
3. flip angle

___ a. 1 only
___ b. 2 only
___ c. 2 and 3 only
___ d. 1, 2, and 3

307. As the static magnetic field strength decreases, how will the T1 of solid matter change?

___ a. shorter
___ b. longer
___ c. stays the same
___ d. depends on the solid matter

308. In solids, local inhomogeneities around the protons are significant and produce which of the following effects?
_____ a. incoherent signal return
_____ b. weak spin-spin interactions
_____ c. rapid spin-spin interactions
_____ d. no effect significant to tissue relaxation

309. Fluids can have a variety of appearances based on

_____.
_____ a. proton structure
_____ b. protein content
_____ c. electron configuration
_____ d. molecular weight

310. The ratio of the amplitude of the signal received to the average amplitude of the noise is called _____.
_____ a. contrast-to-noise ratio
_____ b. signal average
_____ c. gyromagnetic ratio
_____ d. SNR ratio

311. Which of the following statements is true?
1. Noise is not constant for each patient.
2. Noise depends on the build of the patient and the area under examination and the inherent noise of the system.
3. Noise occurs at all frequencies and is also random in time.
_____ a. 1 only
_____ b. 2 only
_____ c. 1 and 3 only
_____ d. 2 and 3 only

312. Which of the parameters below will affect SNR?
    1. TR, TE, and flip angle
    2. proton density of the FOV
    3. voxel volume

    ___ a. 1 only
    ___ b. 2 only
    ___ c. 1 and 3 only
    ___ d. 1, 2, and 3

313. A volume of tissue within the patient is determined by what factors?
    ___ a. the pixel area and the voxel size
    ___ b. the pixel size and the pulse sequence
    ___ c. the slice thickness and the voxel size
    ___ d. the slice thickness and the pixel size

314. What effect will doubling the FOV have on SNR?
    ___ a. doubles SNR
    ___ b. triples SNR
    ___ c. halves SNR
    ___ d. quadruples SNR

315. How many times is the phase encoding gradient turned on to acquire each image for a SE pulse sequence using a TR of 2500 msec, a TE of 35 msec, a matrix of 256 by 256, a FOV of 24 cm, and a NEX of 2?
    ___ a. 256
    ___ b. 512
    ___ c. 1024
    ___ d. 2500

316. What is the term used to describe the degree to which the substance becomes magnetized or the ratio of the applied

magnetization to the resultant magnetic field of the substance?

___ a. magnetization

___ b. transverse magnetization

___ c. magnetic susceptibility

___ d. magnetism

317. The slice thickness, collected by using a range of frequencies in the RF pulse, is called _____.

___ a. pulse profile

___ b. sampling time

___ c. sample rate

___ d. transmit bandwidth

318. Receive or image bandwidth is inversely proportional to which of the following?

___ a. sampling rate

___ b. sampling time

___ c. duty cycle

___ d. all of the above

319. TR has a direct effect on which of the parameters below?

___ a. slice thickness

___ b. sample rate

___ c. acquisition time

___ d. sample time

320. SNR can be improved by which of the following?

___ a. increasing the pixel size

___ b. increasing the acquisition time

___ c. decreasing the RF range

___ d. all of the above

321. The TR, when scanning using ECG triggering, is determined by:
   ___ a. the length of time the frequency gradient is applied
   ___ b. the patient's heart rate
   ___ c. the sample time
   ___ d. the radiologist

322. In an IR pulse sequence, TI (time of inversion), should be in what relation to the rest of the pulse sequence to create heavily T1-weighted images?
   ___ a. 300 msec less than the TR
   ___ b. 1/4 the TR
   ___ c. the T1 of the tissue
   ___ d. follow the 90° RF pulse

323. What effect does increasing the TE have on contrast?
   ___ a. increases the contrast based on T2 relaxation times
   ___ b. reduces the contrast based on T2 relaxation times
   ___ c. reduces the contrast based on T1 relaxation times
   ___ d. a and c

324. When does the presaturation pulse occur in the pulse sequence?
   ___ a. prior to the initial RF pulse
   ___ b. after the initial RF pulse
   ___ c. between the RF pulse and the inverting pulse
   ___ d. it depends on the type of presaturation desired

325. What effect does reducing the TE have on image quality?
    1. increases the contrast based on T2 relaxation times
    2. increases the proton density contrast weighting
    3. reduces contrast based on T2 relaxation times

    ___ a. 2 only
    ___ b. 1 and 2 only
    ___ c. 2 and 3 only
    ___ d. 3 only

326. In IR pulse sequences, the primary contrast controlling mechanism is which of the following?
    ___ a. TR
    ___ b. TR and TI
    ___ c. TI
    ___ d. TR, TE, and TI

327. T1 relaxation time is defined as the length of time for what percentage of the longitudinal magnetization to be recovered?
    ___ a. 63
    ___ b. 68
    ___ c. 69
    ___ d. 100

328. In a GRE pulse sequence what effect does reducing the flip angle while holding the TR constant have on image quality?
    ___ a. reduces T2* weighting
    ___ b. reduces spin density weighting
    ___ c. reduces saturation
    ___ d. reduces scan time

329. The receive bandwidth is related to the slope of which gradient?
    ____ a. frequency encoding or read out gradient
    ____ b. phase encoding gradient
    ____ c. slice-select gradient
    ____ d. all of the above

330. What effect does decreasing the receive bandwidth have on SNR?
    ____ a. decreases it
    ____ b. inverts it
    ____ c. increases it
    ____ d. has no relation or effect on it

331. Variations in the slice thickness can be controlled by which factors?
    1. transmit bandwidth
    2. gradient amplitude
    3. sample rate

    ____ a. 1 only
    ____ b. 2 only
    ____ c. 1 and 2 only
    ____ d. 2 and 3 only

332. What effect does reducing the receive bandwidth have on the length of time the frequency encoding gradient is on?
    ____ a. increases time
    ____ b. decreases time
    ____ c. has no effect on time
    ____ d. is directly proportional to it

333. Reducing the FOV by a factor of 2 has what effect on the voxel volume?
    ____ a. reduces it by the $\sqrt{2}$
    ____ b. reduces it by a factor of 2
    ____ c. reduces it by a factor of 4
    ____ d. reduces it by a factor of 8

334. The total amount of time required for each view or phase encoding step in image formation is called _____.
    1. TR
    2. duty cycle
    3. tau

    ___ a. 1 only
    ___ b. 2 only
    ___ c. 1 and 2
    ___ d. 1 and 3

335. If the TR of a GRE pulse sequence is less than T2 (and T2*), what condition exists?
    ___ a. spin rephasing
    ___ b. saturation
    ___ c. steady state
    ___ d. equilibrium

336. In STIR pulse sequences, the TI time must be set to what value to suppress the signal from a tissue?
    ___ a. the T1 relaxation time
    ___ b. 69% of the T1 relaxation time
    ___ c. 1/4 the TR time
    ___ d. same as TR time

337. In a fast spin echo (FSE) pulse sequence with an echo train length of 16 echoes, what is the number of k-space lines filled per TR?
    ___ a. 4
    ___ b. 8
    ___ c. 16
    ___ d. 32

338. Which of the following causes an increase in SNR when acquiring 3DFT pulse sequences?
    1. increase in FOV
    2. decrease in TR
    3. increase in slices

    ___ a. 1 only
    ___ b. 1 and 2 only
    ___ c. 1 and 3 only
    ___ d. 1, 2, and 3

339. What is the first moment of flow called?
    ___ a. original position
    ___ b. acceleration
    ___ c. velocity
    ___ d. turbulence

340. What is the second moment of flow called?
    ___ a. original position
    ___ b. acceleration
    ___ c. velocity
    ___ d. turbulence

341. Where in k-space is the effective TE placed when performing FSE pulse sequences?
    ___ a. throughout k-space
    ___ b. in the central lines of k-space
    ___ c. on the outer lines of k-space
    ___ d. it depends on the effective TE

342. Which of the following is not an advantage when performing GRE over SE pulse sequences?
    ___ a. dramatically reduced scan times (due to short TR)
    ___ b. lower RF power deposition
    ___ c. true T2 tissue contrast acquired
    ___ d. increased number of slices per unit time

343. What is the advantage of applying a gradient pulse following the echo and before the next RF pulse?
    1. to spoil the signal in the transverse plane
    2. to make the gradient phase dispersion nonzero
    3. to provide more T1 dependence

    ___ a. 1 only
    ___ b. 1 and 2 only
    ___ c. 2 and 3 only
    ___ d. 1, 2, and 3

344. For short TR values, rephased GRE sequences have which of the following advantages?
    1. preserve transverse signal
    2. both signals contribute to the next RF pulse
    3. increase T2* dependence

    ___ a. 1 only
    ___ b. 1 and 3 only
    ___ c. 2 only
    ___ d. 1, 2, and 3

345. In conventional spin echo (CSE) pulse sequences the scan time is determined by the product of which of the following?
    ___ a. TR, Npe, and NEX
    ___ b. TR, Nslices, and Npe
    ___ c. TR, TE, Npe, and NEX
    ___ d. TR, number of frequency steps, Npe

346. What does echo train length refer to?
    ___ a. the length of time for sampling the echo
    ___ b. the total length of time needed to read out the echo
    ___ c. the number of echoes used per TR to comprise the image
    ___ d. the length of time before the echo is sampled

347. Which of the following statements is true of FSE pulse sequences?
    1. Large signal jumps between echoes create blurring in the image.
    2. The larger the number of echo trains the shorter the scan time.
    3. The larger the number of echo trains the more slices can be acquired.

    ____ a. 1 only
    ____ b. 2 only
    ____ c. 1 and 2 only
    ____ d. 1, 2, and 3

348. Which of the effects below is expected when reducing the echo train spacing (ETS)?
    1. increase in the number of slices allowed
    2. improve the contrast control of the image
    3. reduce blurring

    ____ a. 1 only
    ____ b. 2 only
    ____ c. 2 and 3 only
    ____ d. 1, 2, and 3

349. An additional phase encode function added to a CSE pulse sequence design would be descriptive of what other type of pulse sequence design?
    ____ a. CSE
    ____ b. Rephased SE
    ____ c. Hahn spin echo
    ____ d. 3DFT SE

350. Considering a single tissue, the maximum SNR per unit of scan time occurs at a TR of what value?
    ____ a. TR of 3 times the T1
    ____ b. TR of 4 times the T1
    ____ c. TR of 1.26 times the T1
    ____ d. TR equal to the T1

351. At what flip angle is the maximum transverse magnetization obtained?

___ a. 45°

___ b. 90°

___ c. 180°

___ d. 360°

352. What is the purpose of the 180° RF pulse following the 90° RF pulse in an SE pulse sequence?

___ a. to cause the spins to go to an even higher energy state

___ b. to provide for increased longitudinal magnetization

___ c. to assure longitudinal magnetization

___ d. to reverse the direction and rephase the net magnetization vector

353. The contrast produced during a CSE pulse sequence using a short TR and short TE produces _____ type of image contrast.

___ a. T1-weighted

___ b. T2-weighted

___ c. T2*-weighted

___ d. PD-weighted

354. As the FOV is decreased, why does spatial resolution increase?

1. pixel size is reduced
2. matrix size is reduced
3. SNR is increased

___ a. 1 only

___ b. 1 and 2 only

___ c. 2 only

___ d. 1, 2, and 3

355. A pulse sequence that uses a TR of 1800 msec, a TE of 30 msec and a TI of 110 msec produces _____ type of contrast.
    ____ a. T1-weighted
    ____ b. T1-weighted fat suppression
    ____ c. T2*-weighted
    ____ d. PD-weighted

356. A pulse sequence that starts with a 90° RF pulse and is followed by at least one 180° RF pulse is characterized as _____ type of pulse sequence?
    ____ a. IR
    ____ b. GRE
    ____ c. CSE
    ____ d. partial saturation

357. In which of the following pulse sequences is the minimum slice thickness not governed by the maximum gradient strength?
    ____ a. FSE
    ____ b. 3DFT
    ____ c. narrow bandwidth pulse sequences
    ____ d. fast gradient recalled echo (fast GRE) pulse sequences

358. Why are gaps often used between image sections?
    1. more coverage
    2. reduce cross-talk
    3. increase SNR

    ____ a. 2 only
    ____ b. 2 and 3 only
    ____ c. 3 only
    ____ d. 1, 2, and 3

359. Which of the choices below creates images with the strongest signal if the proton densities of the tissues are nearly equal?

____ a. long T1 times

____ b. increased Brownian motion

____ c. long T2 times

____ d. tissues with increased flow

360. To achieve thin slices, a steep slice-select gradient slope and/or what type of transmit bandwidth is applied?

____ a. broad

____ b. narrow

____ c. frequency

____ d. receive

361. The steepness of the slope of the gradient determines the size of the anatomy displayed along the frequency axis. What is this region called?

____ a. receive bandwidth

____ b. diameter spherical volume

____ c. FOV

____ d. frequency axis

362. What is the duration of the frequency-encoding gradient during readout called?

____ a. duty cycle

____ b. echo time

____ c. sample rate

____ d. sample time

363. The Nyquist theorem states that any signal must be sampled how many times per cycle to represent or reproduce it accurately?

____ a. once

____ b. four times

____ c. at least twice

____ d. at least four times

364. What is the sampling time inversely proportional to?
    1. sampling rate
    2. receive bandwidth
    3. transmit bandwidth

    ___ a. 1 only
    ___ b. 1 and 2 only
    ___ c. 3 only
    ___ d. 1 and 3

365. To achieve thick slices, shallow slice-select gradient slope and/or what type of transmit bandwidth is applied?
    ___ a. broad
    ___ b. narrow
    ___ c. frequency
    ___ d. receive

366. What is the time between successive RF pulses applied to the same slice called?
    ___ a. tau
    ___ b. NEX
    ___ c. TR
    ___ d. T1

367. The number of phase encoding and frequency-encoding steps used to create the image is called _____.
    ___ a. an acquisition
    ___ b. matrix
    ___ c. FOV
    ___ d. resolution

368. What is the major determinant of signal within the image?
    ___ a. T1 and T2 tissue characteristics
    ___ b. the pulse sequence
    ___ c. the proton density
    ___ d. the RF power level

369. If a flowing nucleus is adjacent to a stationary nucleus in a voxel, there will be a phase difference between the two nuclei that causes _____.

  ____ a. signal increase
  ____ b. intravoxel dephasing
  ____ c. signal void
  ____ d. counterflow

370. If the original receiver bandwidth is 8 kHz and the new receiver bandwidth is 4 kHz, what percentage increase or decrease in SNR results?

  ____ a. 20% increase
  ____ b. 40% increase
  ____ c. 20% decrease
  ____ d. 40% decrease

371. If the FOV is decreased from 36 cm to 18 cm, what is the necessary increase in scan time (NEX) to obtain an equivalent SNR?

  ____ a. 4 times
  ____ b. 6 times
  ____ c. 8 times
  ____ d. 16 times

372. What percentage of the SNR remains if the matrix size is reduced from 256 to 192, all other parameters remaining the same?

  ____ a. 66%
  ____ b. 71%
  ____ c. 75%
  ____ d. 87%

373. What is the sample rate proportional to?
    1. sample time
    2. receive bandwidth
    3. transmit bandwidth

    ____ a. 1 only
    ____ b. 1 and 2
    ____ c. 2 only
    ____ d. 1 and 3

374. SNR is proportional to both voxel volume and

    _____.

    ____ a. sampling rate
    ____ b. any parameter that alters the size of the voxel
    ____ c. receive bandwidth
    ____ d. phase encoding steps

375. What percentage of signal-to-noise remains when the matrix size is reduced from 256 to 128?

    ____ a. 66
    ____ b. 71
    ____ c. 75
    ____ d. 87

376. What effect does lengthening the TE have on SNR?

    ____ a. increase it
    ____ b. decrease it
    ____ c. no effect
    ____ d. it depends on the TR

377. The time from the initial RF pulse to the middle of the listening window is called?

    ____ a. TR
    ____ b. tau
    ____ c. TE
    ____ d. duty cycle

378. Which of the following determines the amount of gap necessary to minimize cross-talk and signal degradation?
    ____ a. transmit bandwidth
    ____ b. RF pulse waveform
    ____ c. sample time
    ____ d. sample rate

379. If the sampling rate is decreased while the number of samples remains, what happens to the total sampling time or acquisition window?
    ____ a. increase
    ____ b. decrease
    ____ c. no effect
    ____ d. it depends on the bandwidth

380. An image acquired using a TR of 2500 msec and a TE of 90 msec produces _____ type of image contrast.
    ____ a. T1-weighted
    ____ b. T2-weighted
    ____ c. T2*-weighted
    ____ d. PD-weighted

381. An image acquisition where one line of k-space for slice one is filled and then the same line of k-space is filled for slice two is representative of which type of image acquisition?
    ____ a. sequential
    ____ b. 2D volumetric
    ____ c. 3D volumetric
    ____ d. multiecho

382. From the following parameters what will the scan time be, in minutes, to acquire the data?

TR	2000 msec	Frequency steps	256
TE	60 msec	NEX	2
T1	800 msec	Flip angle	90°
Pixel size	.95 x .95 mm	Phase steps	192

     a. 6.4 min
     b. 12.8 min
     c. 17.06 min
     d. 25.6 min

383. Which of the following events would be appropriate to acquire a true T2-weighted image?

     a. 23° RF followed by a 180° RF pulse
     b. 90° RF followed by a gradient reversal
     c. 25° RF pulse followed by a gradient reversal
     d. 90° RF pulse followed by a 180° RF pulse

384. If the TR is increased when acquiring rapid or FSE images which of the following would be expected?

1. increase in T2-weighting
2. increase in the number of slices
3. decrease in motion artifacts

     a. 1 only
     b. 2 only
     c. 1 and 2 only
     d. 1, 2, and 3

385. What is the main contrast controlling mechanism or parameter when acquiring fast GRE pulse sequence images?

     a. TR
     b. TE
     c. TI
     d. flip angle

386. In which of the pulse sequences below is all of the image information collected with each inversion pulse as opposed to one line of data per pulse?

    ____ a. IR

    ____ b. fast GRE

    ____ c. STIR

    ____ d. none of the above

387. Calculate the pixel size for a 24-cm FOV and a 256 x 256 image matrix.

    ____ a. .094 mm

    ____ b. .94 mm

    ____ c. 6.1 mm

    ____ d. 10.6 mm

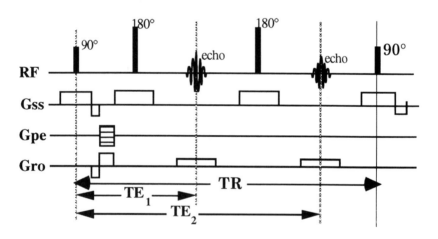

Figure 24

388. How would you characterize the pulse sequence in Figure 24?

    ____ a. SE single echo

    ____ b. FSE double echo

    ____ c. CSE double echo

    ____ d. GRE double echo

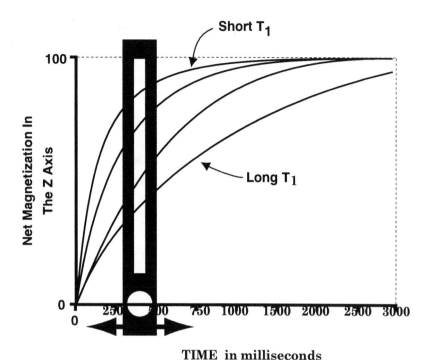

Figure 25

389. An image acquired in the range of TR indicated by the slider in Figure 25 would produce images with _____ type of contrast.

    ___ a. T1-weighted
    ___ b. T2-weighted
    ___ c. PD-weighted
    ___ d. T2*-weighted

390. In 3D imaging, slices are created using which of the processes below?

_____ a. each slice is excited individually creating separate precessional frequencies for slice locations

_____ b. different RF pulses are used to select the individual slice locations

_____ c. the slice-select gradient is turned on for as many times as there are slices

_____ d. the phase-encoding gradient is used to cause phase shifts separating the individual slices from one another

391. In k-space one region or direction represents phase while the other direction represents what process?

_____ a. gradient direction

_____ b. slice thickness

_____ c. amplitude

_____ d. frequency

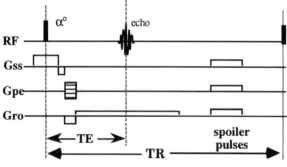

α = partial flip angle

Figure 26

392. What type of pulse sequence is characterized by the series of events as shown in Figure 26?
 ___ a. SE single echo
 ___ b. IR
 ___ c. rephased GRE
 ___ d. spoiled GRE

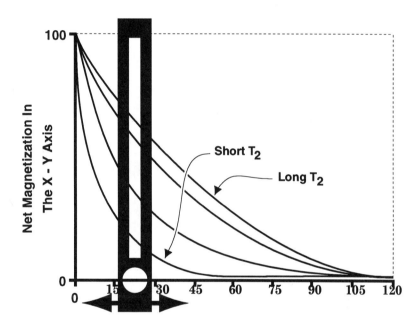

Time Milliseconds

Figure 27

393. Images acquired in the region of the scaler in Figure 27 would create image contrast of which type?
 ___ a. T1-weighted
 ___ b. T2-weighted
 ___ c. PD-weighted
 ___ d. T2* -weighted

394. Which of the parameters below, if increased, causes an increase in SNR for 3D sequences?
    1. FOV
    2. TE
    3. number of slices

    ___ a. 1 only
    ___ b. 1 and 2 only
    ___ c. 1 and 3 only
    ___ d. 1, 2, and 3

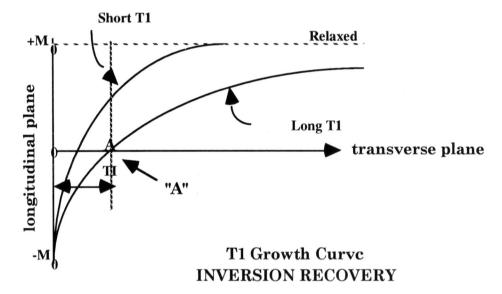

Figure 28

395. What is the area depicted as "A" on the graph in Figure 28, where the net magnetization intersects the transverse plane as the tissues return to the longitudinal magnetization?

    ___ a. short T1 relaxation
    ___ b. transverse magnetization
    ___ c. null point
    ___ d. T2 relaxation time

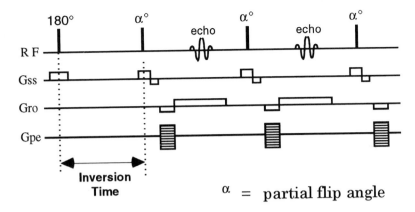

Figure 29

396. What type of pulse sequence is characterized in Figure 29?

_____ a. IR

_____ b. STIR

_____ c. fast GRE

_____ d. inversion gradient echo

397. What substances are used to create the static magnetic field in a superconductive magnet?

____ a. iron, platinum
____ b. niobium, titanium
____ c. aluminum, stainless steel
____ d. neodymium, barium

398. Which of these do not describe a substance's response to a magnetic field?

____ a. paramagnetism
____ b. pyromagnetism
____ c. diamagnetism
____ d. ferromagnetism

399. According to Faraday's law of induction, _____ will generate a voltage and current in a conductor?

____ a. a changing RF pulse
____ b. a changing oscillating magnetic field
____ c. a changing magnetic field
____ d. a changing net magnetic vector

400. Which of these groups contain a substance that is not paramagnetic?

1. platinum, iridium, gadolinium
2. iridium, magnesium, gadolinium
3. platinum, iridium, manganese

____ a. 1 and 2 only
____ b. 2 only
____ c. 1 and 3 only
____ d. 1, 2, and 3

401. Which of these groups contain a substance that is not fer-romagnetic?
  1. iron, cobalt, nickel
  2. iron, nickel, gold
  3. cobalt, nickel, zinc

  ___ a. 1 and 2 only
  ___ b. 2 only
  ___ c. 2 and 3 only
  ___ d. 1, 2, and 3

402. The apparent magnetism of an atom can be shown by the following equation: $B = H_0(1+x)$. When is a substance paramagnetic?

  ___ a. $x < 0$
  ___ b. $x > 0$
  ___ c. $x = 0$
  ___ d. $x \geq 0$

403. One gauss is the strength of the magnetic field measured 1 cm from a straight wire that carries _____ of cur-rent.

  ___ a. one volt (1 V)
  ___ b. five volts (5 V)
  ___ c. one amp (1 A)
  ___ d. five amps (5 A)

404. Which of these magnet types is not capable of producing a vertical static magnetic field?
  1. permanent
  2. iron-core resistive
  3. superconductive
  4. air-core resistive

  ___ a. 1 only
  ___ b. 2 and 4 only
  ___ c. 3 only
  ___ d. 3 and 4 only

405. A factor that governs the efficiency of the passage of current is the inherent resistance of the coil. Which law is used to determine the degree of resistance along a wire?

   _____   a. Faraday's law

   _____   b. Tesla's law

   _____   c. Ohm's law

   _____   d. Helmholtz's law

406. Niobium and titanium and alloys are materials used to create the superconductive magnet. The materials become superconductive at what temperature?

   _____   a. $0°$ K

   _____   b. $10°$ K

   _____   c. $0°$ C

   _____   d. $5°$ C

407. When shimming the static magnetic field, the homogeneity of the magnetic field for clinical imaging purposes is 10 ppm. What is the homogeneity requirement for spectroscopic procedures?

   _____   a. .5 ppm

   _____   b. 1 ppm

   _____   c. 5 ppm

   _____   d. 10 ppm

408. Which of these is the magnetic field strength proportional to?

   _____   a. the amount of current passed through the loops of wire

   _____   b. the number and size of the loops

   _____   c. how closely the loops are spaced

   _____   d. all of the above

409. What does the magnitude of the current passing through the gradient coil determine?
___ a. the strength of the gradient
___ b. the gradient slope
___ c. the direction of the gradient field
___ d. the length of the gradient field

410. According to Faraday's law, the component of the magnetization in the _____ plane induces a current in RF receiver coils.
___ a. longitudinal
___ b. scan
___ c. transverse
___ d. orthogonal

411. What does the degree of magnetism exhibited by a particular substance depend on?
___ a. the number of protons and neutrons in the nucleus
___ b. the electron configuration
___ c. the magnetic susceptibility of the atoms
___ d. b and c

412. Most iron core resistive magnets use what type of RF coil design?
___ a. Helmholtz
___ b. solenoidal
___ c. bird cage
___ d. saddle-shape

413. What determines the magnetic susceptibility response to an externally applied magnetic field?
___ a. the nuclear characteristics of the atom
___ b. the electron configuration of the atom
___ c. the number of protons within the nucleus
___ d. all of the above

414. Saddle-shaped RF coils can be used with which type of magnet design?
    1. air-core resistive magnets
    2. superconductive magnets
    3. permanent magnets

    ____ a. 1 only
    ____ b. 1 and 2 only
    ____ c. 2 only
    ____ d. 1, 2, 3

415. What is the unique advantage of phased array coils?
    ____ a. They are several receive coils linked to one receive channel.
    ____ b. They are one large receive coil with several receive channels.
    ____ c. They are several receive coils each with a different receive channel.
    ____ d. They provide higher SNR because of their combined receive channel design.

416. This coil has a characteristic drop-off in signal, $(1/r^2)$, beyond the physical edge of the coil.
    ____ a. quadrature
    ____ b. Helmholtz pair
    ____ c. planar surface
    ____ d. saddle-shaped

417. What is the "Q" of a coil?
    ____ a. the quantity of closely spaced loops that create the coil
    ____ b. the quotient or diameter of the coil
    ____ c. the quantity or rate of drop off of the signal 1 cm from the center of the coil
    ____ d. the quality factor for the coil loaded with a patient

418. Why must the center frequency be adjusted prior to routine scanning?

___ a. To determine the amount of RF power required to flip the net magnetization into the transverse plane.

___ b. To determine the correct impedance of the receive coil.

___ c. To determine and match the exact frequency that the protons are precessing within the center of the magnetic field.

___ d. To determine the amount of signal amplification needed to receive a strong enough signal from the patient.

419. What procedures are carried out during "prescan"?

___ a. tuning coils, setting center frequency

___ b. tuning coils, setting center frequency, adjusting transmit attenuation

___ c. tuning coils, setting center frequency, adjusting transmit and receive attenuation

___ d. tuning coils, adjusting transmit and receive attenuation

420. What is the potential SNR gain when using quadrature coils vs. linearly polarized coils.

___ a. 1/2

___ b. $\sqrt{2}$

___ c. 2

___ d. 4

421. Real and imaginary are defined as components of the total signal that are phase shifted _____ and compared with the reference RF oscillator within the scanner.

___ a. horizontally and transverse

___ b. 0° and 90°

___ c. 90° and 180°

___ d. 0° and 180°

422. What does the transmit attenuation adjust to generate the appropriate B1 magnetic field?

____ a. voltage and current

____ b. radio frequency

____ c. receiver gain

____ d. none of the above

423. For optimal system performance at various RFs, the impedance of the transmit/receive coil must be matched to _____?

____ a. the power amplification induced by the body

____ b. the impedance of the transmission line

____ c. RF amplifier

____ d. magnetic field strength

424. Which of these are a benefit for using phased array coils?

1. use of small surface coils for increased SNR and resolution
2. increase longitudinal coverage
3. increase uniformity across a whole volume

____ a. 1 only

____ b. 1 and 2 only

____ c. 2 only

____ d. 1, 2, and 3

425. Which of these is not true of phase array coils?

1. The signal output from each coil is separately received.
2. All the data can be acquired in a single sequence.
3. Each individual coil receives signal from all coils.

____ a. 1 and 2 only

____ b. 2 and 3 only

____ c. 3 only

____ d. 1, 2, and 3

426. Which of these RF coils is designed to be used with a vertical magnetic field?
    1. volume coil
    2. surface coil
    3. solenoidal coils
    4. saddle-shaped coils

    ____ a. 1 and 3 only
    ____ b. 3 only
    ____ c. 1, 2, and 3 only
    ____ d. all of the above

427. A gradient coil, when active, causes the following result on the main magnetic field:

    ____ a. The field becomes stronger from one end and weaker at the other.
    ____ b. The field becomes increasingly stronger from isocenter.
    ____ c. The field becomes increasingly weaker from iso-center.
    ____ d. The field becomes stronger throughout the main magnetic field.

428. What are the benefits of using steeper gradients?
    1. minimizes field inhomogeneities
    2. reduces chemical shift errors
    3. produces high amplitude signals

    ____ a. 1 only
    ____ b. 1 and 2 only
    ____ c. 3 only
    ____ d. 1, 2, and 3

429. What is the term called when the nonrectangular RF pulse profile of one slice causes stimulation and therefore contamination of an adjacent slice?
    ___ a. nonsinc pulse waveform
    ___ b. cross-talk
    ___ c. eddy currents
    ___ d. dephasing

430. What is the unit of measurement for the strength of the gradient magnetic field?
    ___ a. W/kg
    ___ b. mHz/cm
    ___ c. mT/m
    ___ d. mHz/G

431. Increasing the amplitude of the slice-select gradient causes the following result if the transmit bandwidth remains constant:
    ___ a. greater signal return
    ___ b. an increase in slice thickness
    ___ c. a different slice orientation
    ___ d. a decrease in slice thickness

432. Which of the following fat suppression methods uses a short-duration RF pulse that rotates the fat magnetization into the transverse plane and then dephases it using a spoiler gradient?
    ___ a. phase evolution, Dixon method
    ___ b. frequency-selective excitation (fat sat)
    ___ c. T1-dependent suppression
    ___ d. Selective water excitation, slice-selective gradient reversal

433. In which gradient do the phase dispersions not equal zero during the collection of the echo?

_____ a. slice-select gradient

_____ b. phase-encoding gradient

_____ c. frequency-encoding gradient

_____ d. all of the above

434. The slice-select gradient must be turned on during which of the following events of a SE pulse sequence?

1. initial excitation of the slice
2. 180° refocusing of the spins
3. readout of the signal or echo

_____ a. 1 only

_____ b. 2 only

_____ c. 1 and 2 only

_____ d. 1, 2, and 3

435. What is the gradient rise time?

_____ a. the time it takes to turn on the gradient once the scan has been initiated

_____ b. the time it takes to ramp the gradient to full strength

_____ c. a measure of the gradient's maximum field strength capacity

_____ d. shorter for echo planar imaging vs. routine imaging

436. What is the maximum gradient amplitude for most MR scanners?

_____ a. .1 mT/m

_____ b. .5 mT/m

_____ c. 5 mT/m

_____ d. 10 mT/m

437. Which of these statements is not true about gradients?

____ a. When on, the magnetic field strength either sub-tracts from or adds to B_0

____ b. The slope of the resulting magnetic field is the amplitude of the magnetic field gradient

____ c. Steep gradient slopes alter the magnetic field strength between two points less than shallow gradient slopes

____ d. The slope determines the rate of change of the magnetic field strength along the gradient axis

438. Which gradient is used to alter the magnetic field strength and thus precessional frequency to select sagittal slices?

____ a. z-gradient

____ b. x-gradient

____ c. y-gradient

____ d. none of the above

439. Applying two gradients simultaneously would be helpful in only which of the following imaging processes?

____ a. no phase wrap

____ b. oblique slice acquisition

____ c. reducing eddy currents in the magnet

____ d. gradient reversal

440. Referencing transaxial images, if the x-direction is used for frequency encoding, which gradient is used for phase encoding?

____ a. x-gradient

____ b. y-gradient

____ c. z-gradient

____ d. none of the above

441. If a proton moves across a gradient of increasing strength, what would happen to its precession?

       a. it would dephase

       b. it would not be affected

       c. it would accelerate

       d. it would stop

Fundamentals of Image Formation

442. What type of magnetism is the RF receive coil able to measure directly?
    1. longitudinal
    2. transverse
    3. gradient

    ____ a. 1 and 2 only
    ____ b. 1 only
    ____ c. 2 only
    ____ d. 1, 2, and 3

443. What is the wobbling motion of the nucleus as it spins about the magnetic field called?
    ____ a. resonance
    ____ b. relaxation
    ____ c. precession
    ____ d. net magnetism

444. What is the precessional frequency of hydrogen exposed to a .5 T magnetic field?
    ____ a. 12.31 mHz
    ____ b. 21.29 mHz
    ____ c. 24.58 mHz
    ____ d. 42.58 mHz

445. The static magnetic field is directly proportional to what?
    ____ a. precessional frequency
    ____ b. gyromagnetic ratio
    ____ c. gradient magnetic field
    ____ d. T2 relaxation time

446. Prior to entering the main magnetic field, why is the patient's net magnetism zero?

    ____ a. Because the main magnetic field frees up the bound hydrogen atoms

    ____ b. Because the spins of the hydrogen atoms are randomly aligned

    ____ c. Because the patient must be exposed to a magnetic field for a minimum of five minutes before their magnetism can be measured

    ____ d. Because the nucleus does not spin until a magnetic field has been applied

447. What is the kG equivalent of a magnetic field strength of 1 T?

    ____ a. 10

    ____ b. 100

    ____ c. 1000

    ____ d. 10,000

448. What two characteristic components must a vector have?

    ____ a. mass, charge

    ____ b. amount, speed

    ____ c. magnitude, direction

    ____ d. energy, speed

449. What is the formula that describes the relationship between the precessional frequency and the applied magnetic field of atoms?

    ____ a. Nyquist theorem

    ____ b. Larmor equation

    ____ c. Bloch equation

    ____ d. Ohm's law

450. Which of these do not represent the Larmor equation?

    1. magnetic field = precessional frequency/gyromagnetic ratio

    2. magnetic field/precessional frequency = gyromagnetic ratio

    3. precessional frequency = gyromagnetic ratio x magnetic field

    ____ a. 1 only

    ____ b. 2 only

    ____ c. 1 and 2 only

    ____ d. 3 only

451. The force of attraction an object experiences when exposed to a magnetic field depends on which of the following factors?

    ____ a. the mass of the object

    ____ b. the ferromagnetic properties of the object

    ____ c. the field strength and rate of change in field strength over distance

    ____ d. all of the above

452. When hydrogen atoms are exposed to a strong homogeneous magnetic field, they have a tendency to do which of the following?

    ____ a. align perpendicular to the magnetic field

    ____ b. all align parallel to the magnetic field

    ____ c. slightly more than half align parallel and the remaining align antiparallel

    ____ d. equal amounts align parallel and antiparallel until the application of the RF pulse

453. An NMR signal can be created from which form of hydrogen?

    ____ a. hydrogen in water

    ____ b. hydrogen in fat

    ____ c. mobile hydrogen protons

    ____ d. all of the above

454. In a homogeneous magnetic field, what rate of precession does hydrogen in water have compared with hydrogen in fat?

    ____ a. hydrogen in water precesses faster than hydrogen in fat

    ____ b. hydrogen in water precesses slower than hydrogen in fat

    ____ c. water and fat hydrogen have equal precessional frequencies

    ____ d. it depends on the magnetic field strength

455. What is the atomic number for the hydrogen atom used to create the NMR signal?

    ____ a. 1

    ____ b. 2

    ____ c. 6

    ____ d. depends on the molecular structure

456. How do small molecules with a higher rate of molecular motion affect T1 relaxation?

    ____ a. They are efficient at returning energy and cause short T1 relaxation times

    ____ b. They are inefficient at returning energy and have a long T1 relaxation time

    ____ c. The size of the molecule does not affect T1 relaxation

    ____ d. They are inefficient at returning energy and have a short T1 relaxation time

457. What interaction does dipole-dipole magnetic interaction refer to?

    1. a proton and an electron
    2. protons
    3. molecules

    ____ a. 1 only

    ____ b. 2 only

    ____ c. 1 and 2 only

    ____ d. 2 and 3 only

458. What is the absorption and re-emission of RF energy by the tissues within the patient called?

____ a. precession

____ b. resonance

____ c. longitudinal relaxation

____ d. transverse relaxation

459. What would be the result if a volume of protons in a magnetic field were suddenly exposed to a graduated magnetic field?

1. The protons would begin to precess at the new magnetic field strength(s).
2. Dephasing of the volume would occur and there would be a range of precessional frequencies.
3. The volume would maintain phase coherency and would begin to precess at the new precessional frequency.

____ a. 1 only

____ b. 2 only

____ c. 1 and 2 only

____ d. 1 and 3 only

460. What must occur to cause protons within a specific volume to absorb RF energy and re-emit it as an NMR signal?

1. The RF energy applied must match the precessional frequency of the protons at that magnetic field strength.
2. The RF energy must be applied perpendicular to the magnetic field.
3. Enough power or energy must be used to tip the net magnetization vector into the transverse plane.

____ a. 1 only

____ b. 1 and 3 only

____ c. 1 and 2 only

____ d. 1, 2, and 3

461. What would be the precessional frequency of hydrogen in a 640 G magnetic field?

_____ a. .2725 mHz

_____ b. 2.725 mHz

_____ c. 27.25 mHz

_____ d. 272.5 mHz

462. What flip angle would be necessary to return the spin system back to its original starting position or state after being excited?

_____ a. 180°

_____ b. 270°

_____ c. 360°

_____ d. 720°

463. To maximize signal return for a given tissue the flip angle depends on the sequence type. For sequences in which no steady state is established, when is the MR signal maximized?

_____ a. at the T1 relaxation

_____ b. at the Ernst angle

_____ c. at the T1 and T2 relaxation

_____ d. at 90°

464. If the net magnetization vector M_z is flipped into the transverse plane by a partial flip RF pulse, what would be the expected result?

_____ a. The signal will be lower than if a 90° flip angle were used.

_____ b. The signal will be higher than if a 90° flip angle were used.

_____ c. The signal will be composed of only longitudinal magnetization.

_____ d. The signal will be dependent on M_z and the fraction of M_z flipped into the transverse plane

465. If only a single RF pulse were applied, what flip angle would produce the optimal signal return?

   ____ a. 10°

   ____ b. 45°

   ____ c. 90°

   ____ d. 180°

466. Which method of disrupting the transverse magnetization coherence does not generate eddy currents and is spatially invariant?

   1. gradient spoiling
   2. RF spoiling
   3. rephased GRE

   ____ a. 1 only

   ____ b. 2 only

   ____ c. 1 and 2 only

   ____ d. 1, 2, and 3

467. What is the term for the range of radiofrequencies in the transmit RF pulse?

   ____ a. sample rate

   ____ b. duty cycle

   ____ c. pulse duration

   ____ d. transmit bandwidth

468. What is the gyromagnetic ratio of the hydrogen atom (H+)?

   ____ a. 42.3759 mHz/T

   ____ b. 42.5759 mHz/T

   ____ c. 43.7559 mHz/T

   ____ d. 47.5259 mHz/T

469. Which of these would potentially generate the most eddy currents?

   ____ a. A heavily T2-weighted SE pulse sequence
   ____ b. A gradient echo using a partial flip angle of less than 25°
   ____ c. A pulse sequence that uses half-Fourier or fractional-NEX imaging
   ____ d. A rapid or fast GRE pulse sequence

470. Which nuclear characteristic causes atoms to create angular momentum?

   ____ a. odd number of electrons
   ____ b. odd number of protons and/or neutrons
   ____ c. odd number of protons and electrons
   ____ d. odd number of protons

471. What factors affect the rate of molecular motion?

   1. molecular size
   2. protein binding effects
   3. how efficiently energy is distributed back to the lattice

   ____ a. 1 only
   ____ b. 1 and 2 only
   ____ c. 1 and 3 only
   ____ d. 1, 2, and 3

472. If the T1 relaxation time of a tissue is 800 msec, approximately how long does it take to recover most of its net longitudinal magnetization (at least 98%)?

   ____ a. 400 msec
   ____ b. 800 msec
   ____ c. 1600 msec
   ____ d. 3200 msec

473. T2 relaxation is the length of time it takes the spin system to lose what percentage of the transverse magnetization?

    _____ a. 37

    _____ b. 63

    _____ c. 98

    _____ d. 100

474. What is another name for thermal relaxation?

    _____ a. spin lattice relaxation

    _____ b. spin-spin relaxation

    _____ c. spin density relaxation

    _____ d. none of the above

475. Which type of RF coil is much more efficient in the transfer of RF power to the patient?

    _____ a. volume coils

    _____ b. phased array coils

    _____ c. quadrature coils

    _____ d. linearly polarized coils

476. Which of these statements is not true?

    _____ a. T1 relaxation increases with increasing field strengths.

    _____ b. T2 relaxation increases with increasing field strengths.

    _____ c. T2 relaxation remains unchanged with increasing field strengths.

    _____ d. T2* relaxation results principally from inhomogeneities in the main magnetic field.

477. Why does fat have a short T1 relaxation time?
   1. Fat is a large molecule that has a lower molecular motion.
   2. Fat does not contain proteins that lower the frequencies.
   3. Long-chain fatty acids tumble at lower frequencies.

   ___ a. 2 only
   ___ b. 1 and 2 only
   ___ c. 1 and 3 only
   ___ d. 1, 2, and 3

478. Pure water has which of the following tissue characteristics?

   ___ a. short T1, short T2
   ___ b. short T1, long T2
   ___ c. long T1, short T2
   ___ d. long T1, long T2

479. Which type of magnetism has its maximum amplitude immediately following the RF pulse?

   ___ a. longitudinal magnetization
   ___ b. transverse magnetization
   ___ c. proton density
   ___ d. all of the above

480. In which type of receive coil are two separate signals being recorded with a potential SNR gain of 2?
   1. circularly polarized
   2. quadrature
   3. linearly polarized

   ___ a. 1 only
   ___ b. 2 only
   ___ c. 1 and 2 only
   ___ d. 2 and 3 only

481. The T1 relaxation value of a tissue is the time required for the tissue's longitudinal magnetization to recover _____ percentage of its equilibrium magnetization.

_____ a. 100

_____ b. 98

_____ c. 63

_____ d. 37

482. What is the interaction called when one proton transfers energy to another proton?

_____ a. spin-spin

_____ b. transfer magnetization

_____ c. spin-lattice

_____ d. cross-talk

483. Which of these flow effects cause an increase in signal intensity?

1. entry phenomenon
2. even echo rephasing
3. diastolic pseudogating

_____ a. 1 only

_____ b. 1 and 2 only

_____ c. 1 and 3 only

_____ d. 1, 2, and 3

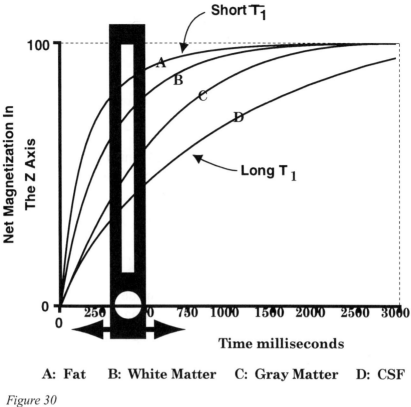

A: Fat   B: White Matter   C: Gray Matter   D: CSF

Figure 30

484. Based on the information in Figure 30, which of the following has the shortest T1 relaxation time?

    ___ a. fat
    ___ b. white matter
    ___ c. gray matter
    ___ d. CSF

485. On a T2-weighted image, why does CSF appear bright?

    ___ a. CSF has a long T1 relaxation time
    ___ b. CSF has a short T1 relaxation time
    ___ c. CSF has a long T2 relaxation time
    ___ d. CSF has a short T2 relaxation time

486. What does the bulk magnetic properties of a substance principally result from?

_____ a. magnetic moments

_____ b. electrons

_____ c. number of protons and neutrons

_____ d. proton density

487. For maximum RF absorption the B1 magnetic field is oriented to _____ the static magnetic field?

_____ a. perpendicular

_____ b. parallel

_____ c. antiparallel

_____ d. adjacent

488. The gradient coils are positioned inside of the main magnet and provide which of the following functions?

1. To linearly distort the main magnetic field
2. To provide spatial variations in the magnetic field for image formation
3. To alter precessional frequencies of protons for spatial encoding

_____ a. 2 only

_____ b. 2 and 3 only

_____ c. 1 and 2 only

_____ d. 1, 2, and 3

489. Slice thickness for a given magnetic field strength is a function of:

1. gradient slope
2. transmit bandwidth
3. sample rate

_____ a. 1 only

_____ b. 2 only

_____ c. 1 and 2 only

_____ d. 1, 2, and 3

490. Typically, gradients are measured in terms of G/cm or mT/m. What does 1 G/cm equal in mT/m?

____ a. .1

____ b. 1

____ c. 10

____ d. 100

491. If a 10 G/cm gradient is applied at the magnet's isocenter, the local magnetic field increases and decreases on either side of isocenter by which of the following amounts?

____ a. 2.5 G

____ b. 5 G

____ c. 10 G

____ d. 20 G

492. During the pulse sequence the slice-select gradient is turned on during which of the following processes?

1. 90° RF pulse
2. 180° RF pulse
3. gradient reversal

____ a. 1 only

____ b. 1 and 2 only

____ c. 1, 2, and 3

____ d. 2 and 3 only

493. To produce a transaxial slice the slice-select gradient is turned on, graduating the magnetic field from:

____ a. superior to inferior

____ b. left to right

____ c. anterior to posterior

____ d. none of the above

494. Two gradients applied at the same time during slice-selection are used to:
    ___ a. reduce eddy currents in the main magnetic field
    ___ b. encode oblique slices
    ___ c. get rid of residual transverse magnetization for steady state precession
    ___ d. encode a 3D volume

495. The spatial encoding process that usually follows the initial RF pulse application is:
    ___ a. slice-selection encoding
    ___ b. phase encoding
    ___ c. frequency encoding
    ___ d. FID

496. Which gradient is applied during slice-selection to excite coronal images?
    ___ a. x-gradient
    ___ b. y-gradient
    ___ c. z-gradient
    ___ d. none of these

497. To create an oblique image oriented at an angle between sagittal and transaxial requires the application of which physical gradients during slice-selection?
    ___ a. x-gradient
    ___ b. z-gradient
    ___ c. x- and z-gradients
    ___ d. x- and y-gradients

498. K-space is a mathematical name for:
    1. raw data
    2. processed data
    3. time domain

    ____ a. 1 only
    ____ b. 2 only
    ____ c. 1 and 2 only
    ____ d. 1 and 3 only

499. Which of these statements is not true regarding k-space?
    ____ a. Individual cells in k-space do not correspond one to one with individual pixels in the MR image
    ____ b. k-space corresponds to the echo data obtained from a single application of the phase encoding gradient
    ____ c. There is no direct correspondence between the location of a cell in k-space and location of a pixel in the image
    ____ d. Rows near the center of the k-space grid correspond to high-order phase encode steps, whereas rows near the top and bottom correspond to lower order phase encodes

500. The frequency-encoding gradient is usually turned on during the readout of the echo and during which other process?
    ____ a. slice-selection
    ____ b. phase encoding
    ____ c. frequency encoding
    ____ d. no other process

501. Where in k-space are the magnetic moments in phase and at the maximum signal amplitude?

_____ a. along the phase encode central reference line

_____ b. along the outer lines of k-space

_____ c. along the frequency encode central reference line

_____ d. along the central reference lines of both phase and frequency-encoding lines

Artifacts

502. An artifact that refers to the differences in resonant frequency of protons due to local differences in chemical environment is called:
    ___ a. truncation artifact
    ___ b. Gibb's artifact
    ___ c. chemical shift
    ___ d. magnetic susceptibility artifact

503. What is the term for the artifact that is caused when two different frequencies with the same peak are placed in the same voxel?
    ___ a. truncation artifact
    ___ b. aliasing artifact
    ___ c. RF discreets
    ___ d. Gibb's artifact

504. Artifacts from motion will appear in which direction?
    ___ a. in the direction of the slice
    ___ b. in the direction of the motion
    ___ c. in the phase encoding direction
    ___ d. in the frequency-encoding direction

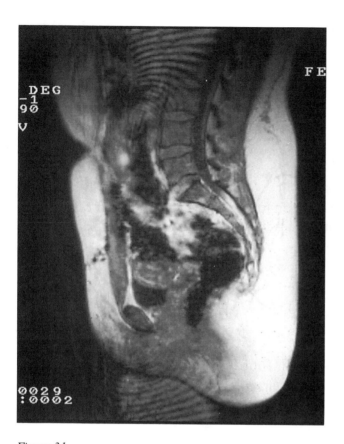

Figure 31

505. What is the artifact called in Figure 31?

_____ a. RF discreets

_____ b. banding

_____ c. aliasing or wraparound

_____ d. static from wool clothing

506. The artifact that appears as multiple rings or bands of regular periodicity or duplication at transitions between high and low intensity signals is termed:

_____ a. truncation

_____ b. aliasing

_____ c. chemical

_____ d. herringbone

507. The actual chemical shift, in Hz, depends on the magnetic field strength. What would the chemical shift be for a 1.0 T field strength?

   _____ a. 42.58 Hz

   _____ b. 149.03 Hz

   _____ c. 223.54 Hz

   _____ d. 298.06 Hz

508. Chemical shift artifacts appear because of which of the following?

   1. Protons in fat and water molecules are separated by a chemical shift of about 3.5 ppm.

   2. The electron configuration of the hydrogen atom is the cause of this phenomenon.

   3. The protons in water will have a lower frequency than protons in fat.

   _____ a. 1 only

   _____ b. 1 and 3 only

   _____ c. 1 and 2 only

   _____ d. 1, 2, and 3

509. Which of these can cause RF interference or RF discreet artifacts?

   1. static electricity

   2. AC current fluctuations

   3. electronic devices

   _____ a. 1 only

   _____ b. 2 and 3 only

   _____ c. 2 only

   _____ d. 1, 2, and 3

510. An artifact that can cause a bright signal at the isocenter or central reference point with a linear dashed pattern along the frequency axis is termed:

____ a. RF discreet

____ b. truncation

____ c. metal

____ d. FID or zero-line

511. The first peak of the RF pulse adjacent to the interface always overshoots the ideal intensity line to a greater degree than subsequent peaks. This can be the cause of what type of artifact?

1. chemical shift
2. Gibb's
3. truncation

____ a. 1 only

____ b. 2 only

____ c. 3 only

____ d. 1 and 2 only

512. An image acquired on a 1.5 T magnet with 256 pixels in the frequency-encoding direction recorded a total receiver bandwidth of 32 kHz. What will be the size of the chemical shift?

____ a. 1.8 pixels

____ b. 3.6 pixels

____ c. 7 pixels

____ d. 18 pixels

513. If the MR signal is sampled less frequently than the Nyquist limit, a misassignment of frequencies can occur and cause _____ artifacts?

____ a. motion

____ b. frequency aliasing

____ c. truncation

____ d. chemical shift

514. Which of these will help to reduce the aliasing artifact?
    1. oversampling
    2. steep bandpass or low pass filter
    3. increasing the number of acquisitions or excitations

    ___ a. 1 only
    ___ b. 1 and 3 only
    ___ c. 1 and 2 only
    ___ d. 1, 2, and 3

515. A light bulb about to go out in an MR scan room could cause _____.
    1. RF artifacts
    2. herringbone artifacts
    3. truncation artifacts

    ___ a. 1 only
    ___ b. 2 only
    ___ c. 1 and 2 only
    ___ d. 1, 2, and 3

516. Gradient moment nulling provides what capability necessary for MR imaging?
    ___ a. gradient rephasing
    ___ b. flow compensation
    ___ c. gradient spoiling
    ___ d. gradient refocusing

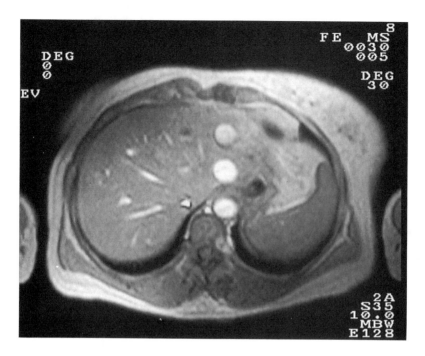

Figure 32

517. What is the most probable cause of the artifact seen in Figure 32?

    ____ a. patient swallowed ping pong balls

    ____ b. unstable gradients

    ____ c. metal artifact on patient

    ____ d. motion artifact from pulsing aorta

518. Chemical shift artifacts, when visible, are always seen:

    1. as a void of signal on the high-frequency side of an organ.

    2. as an addition of signal on the low-frequency side of an organ.

    3. in the frequency encoding direction.

    ____ a. 1 only

    ____ b. 2 only

    ____ c. 1 and 3 only

    ____ d. 1, 2, and 3

519. What is the term for the artifact that appears as multiple rings of regular periodicity or duplication at transitions between high and low intensity signals?

_____ a. chemical shift

_____ b. aliasing

_____ c. truncation

_____ d. magnetic susceptibility

520. A pixel's SNR is proportional to:
    1. the square root of the number of acquisitions(NEX).
    2. the number of phase encoding steps.
    3. the signal within a voxel (voxel volume).

    ____ a. 1 only
    ____ b. 1 and 3 only
    ____ c. 3 only
    ____ d. 1, 2, and 3

521. Which of the following parameter changes causes an increase in spatial resolution?
    1. increasing FOV
    2. increasing matrix size
    3. decreasing the pixel size

    ____ a. 1 only
    ____ b. 2 only
    ____ c. 1 and 2 only
    ____ d. 2 and 3 only

522. All other parameters remaining, if the slice thickness of 10 mm is reduced to 5 mm, to maintain SNR, the number of acquisitions must be increased by a factor of:
    ____ a. .5
    ____ c. 1.41
    ____ b. 2
    ____ d. 4

523. Eddy currents may be induced in which of the following?
    1. the MR magnet
    2. the patient
    3. the cables and wires

    ____ a. 1 only
    ____ b. 1 and 3 only
    ____ c. 2 only
    ____ d. 1, 2, and 3

524. If the slice thickness is reduced, what happens to the image quality if all other parameters remain the same?

   1. partial voluming decreases
   2. signal to noise decreases
   3. spatial resolution increases

    ____ a. 1 only
    ____ b. 1 and 3 only
    ____ c. 1, 2, and 3
    ____ d. none of the above

525. Which of these pulse sequences has a mechanism to minimize the effect of slight inhomogeneities in the magnetic field?

    ____ a. CSE
    ____ b. GRE
    ____ c. partial saturation
    ____ d. none of the above

Post Test

1. Which of the following implants may pose a problem during scanning?
   ___ a. implantable drug infusion pumps
   ___ b. cardiac pacemakers/breast tissue expanders
   ___ c. bone growth stimulators
   ___ d. all of the above

2. Which of the following could result from scanning a patient with a cardiac pacemaker?
   ___ a. changes in the programming
   ___ b. induced current in the lead wire/patient burns
   ___ c. pacemaker may become dislodged and pulled from the patient's chest
   ___ d. a and b

3. Which of the following procedures would be acceptable in checking for ferrous qualities of accessory devices?
   ___ a. check the weight
   ___ b. use a hand-held magnet
   ___ c. manufacturer label
   ___ d. take the device in the room and see if it is attracted

4. A _____ reaction to contrast involves respiratory, cardiovascular, cutaneous, and possibly gastrointestinal manifestations.
   ___ a. superficial
   ___ b. bronchial
   ___ c. anaphylactoid
   ___ d. none of the above

5. Which of the following factors are responsible for inducing a physiologic response to induced voltage?

___ a. orientation of the gradient field

___ b. patient's size

___ c. frequency of stimulus

___ d. all of the above

6. _____ are reported visual sensations, or flashes of light, that result from direct excitation of the optic nerve, induced by the gradient magnetic fields.

___ a. magnetophosphenes

___ b. phosphorescence

___ c. hypermagnetophenes

___ d. none of the above

7. At the present time, which of the following is the FDA recommended safe level for the SAR level to the head?

___ a. 8.0 W/kg

___ b. 0.4 W/kg

___ c. 4 W/kg

___ d. 3.2 W/kg

8. Compared with conventional spin echo sequences, the fast pulse sequences, such as fast spin echo (FSE) or rapid acquisition relaxation enhanced (RARE) have _____ RF deposition.

___ a. decreased

___ b. increased

___ c. the same

___ d. none of the above

9. Anesthesiologists consider the use of _____ to be a standard practice for monitoring when scanning sedated or anesthetized patients.

___ a. sphygmomanometer

___ b. pulse oximeter

___ c. blood pressure cuff

___ d. respiratory belt

10. After injection, paramagnetic contrast agents affect patient tissue in which of the following ways?
    ___ a. decrease T1 relaxation time
    ___ b. decrease T1 and T2 relaxation time
    ___ c. increase T1 relaxation time
    ___ d. increase T2 relaxation time

11. Which of the following contrast agents is an ionic compound?
    ___ a. Magnevist
    ___ b. Prohance
    ___ c. Omniscan
    ___ d. none of the above

12. Following the injection of contrast, which of the following patients are most likely to have a serious reaction?
    ___ a. those with asthma or allergic respiratory disorders
    ___ b. those with a high BUN level
    ___ c. anemic patients
    ___ d. claustrophobics

13. Which position best demonstrates the collateral ligaments of the knee?
    ___ a. axial
    ___ b. sagittal
    ___ c. coronal
    ___ d. none of the above

14. State the major advantage of using a surface coil.
    ___ a. increased resolution
    ___ b. decreased resolution
    ___ c. increased SNR
    ___ d. increased FOV

15. The closer a receiver coil is to the patient, the less RF energy is needed to create transverse magnetization. Which of the following results from this phenomenon?

____ a. reduced SAR to the patient
____ b. increased surface noise
____ c. increased SAR to the patient
____ d. none of the above

16. Which of the following coils is not a transmit and receive coil?

____ a. head coil
____ b. body coil
____ c. TMJ coil
____ d. extremity coil

17. Which of the following coils provide the highest SNR when scanning a TMJ?

____ a. 5" circular coil
____ b. 3" circular coil
____ c. 5 x 11" license plate receive coil
____ d. endorectal coil

18. Which of the following coils yields the high SNR of a sensitive, small surface coil, yet covers a large area?

____ a. body coil
____ b. extremity coil
____ c. 5 x 11" receive coil
____ d. phased array coil

19. Which of the following coils is considered a volume coil, two coils working in tandem, that images both the anterior and posterior portions of anatomy?

____ a. Helmholtz configuration
____ b. Phased array
____ c. Purcell configuration
____ d. none of the above

20. _____ contrast enhancement occurs when the tissue of interest appears darker on images following the administration of contrast.
    ____ a. isometric
    ____ b. negative
    ____ c. positive
    ____ d. none of the above

21. Calculate the amount of contrast that should be administered to a patient who weighs 75 pounds.
    ____ a. 6 cc
    ____ b. 7 cc
    ____ c. 12 cc
    ____ d. 20 cc

22. Describe the amount of contrast that should be administered to a patient weighing 260 pounds.
    ____ a. 25 cc
    ____ b. 24 cc
    ____ c. 20 cc
    ____ d. none of the above

23. List some of the precautions concerning patients who are given gadolinium.
    ____ a. patients with sickle cell anemia
    ____ b. patients in renal failure
    ____ c. pregnant patients
    ____ d. all of the above

24. Which areas normally enhance following the injection of contrast?
    ____ a. choroid plexus
    ____ b. pineal gland
    ____ c. pituitary gland
    ____ d. all of the above

25. If a technologist wants higher resolution on a hip scan, which of the following would he select?

____ a. 256 x 128

____ b. 256 x 160

____ c. 256 x 192

____ d. 256 x 256

26. _____ is an algorithm which creates a 2D projective image from a 3D dataset, using the value of the brightest pixel.

____ a. MIP

____ b. EPI ·

____ c. MRA

____ d. ERA

27. Gadolinium is a _____ product.

____ a. ferromagnetic

____ b. diamagnetic

____ c. paramagnetic

____ d. ferroionic

28. FDA approved oral contrast displays a _____ appearance in the bowel.

____ a. bright T1/dark T2

____ b. dark T1/bright T2

____ c. dark T1/dark T2

____ d. isointense on both T1 and T2

29. Which of the following are important precautions when using a surface coil?

____ a. restricted FOV

____ b. positioning is critical

____ c. the surface coil must be perpendicular to the XY plane.

____ d. all of the above

30. Hemosiderin displays a _____ appearance on T1 and T2 images.
    ___ a. dark
    ___ b. bright
    ___ c. isointense
    ___ d. mottled

31. Which planes have become widely accepted as the standard orientations for viewing the orbit?
    ___ a. transverse/coronal
    ___ b. axial/sagittal
    ___ c. sagittal/coronal
    ___ d. off axis coronals/off axis sagittals

32. The petrous bone and mastoid air cells are _____ because of the _____ signal from dense bone and air.
    ___ a. bright/high
    ___ b. isointense/medium
    ___ c. black/low
    ___ d. none of the above

33. Except for the corpus callosum and fornix, the major white matter tracts of the brain are best demonstrated on the _____ plane.
    ___ a. axial
    ___ b. sagittal
    ___ c. coronal
    ___ d. off axis coronal

34. _____ is a technique in which a complete image is obtained from one selective excitation pulse. This method is an extremely fast method of acquiring an image.
    ___ a. Maximum intensity projection (MIP)
    ___ b. SNR
    ___ c. MRA
    ___ d. Echo planar imagingy (EPI)

35. Which vessel is most superior in orientation in the body?
    ____ a. hepatic vein
    ____ b. portal vein
    ____ c. splenic vein
    ____ d. inferior mesenteric vein

36. The portal vein drains into which of the following?
    ____ a. hepatic vein and liver
    ____ b. inferior mesenteric vein, superior mesenteric vein, and the splenic vein
    ____ c. common iliac veins
    ____ d. inferior vena cava

37. When using a 5" receiver coil, the depth of coverage is approximately _____ inches.
    ____ a. 5
    ____ b. 10
    ____ c. 2.5
    ____ d. 1.25

38. Which of the following make vessels appear bright?
    ____ a. presaturation pulses
    ____ b. fat saturation pulses
    ____ c. gradient moment nulling
    ____ d. none of the above

39. _____ is an imaging technique that relies primarily on flow-related enhancement to distinguish moving spins from stationary spins in creating MR angiograms.
    ____ a. TOF
    ____ b. PC
    ____ c. MIP
    ____ d. DAC

40. Time of Flight (TOF) MRA is sensitive to flow coming into the field of view or imaging volume. Spins in vessels with slow flow can become saturated. 2D TOF is best for areas with slower flow. All of the following ves-

sels exhibit slow flow except _____, which have higher velocity.

____ a. carotids

____ b. venous systems

____ c. intracranial vessels

____ d. peripheral vessels

41. Which of the following uses the velocity differences or phase shifts on moving spins to provide image contrast in flowing vessels ?

____ a. 2D phase contrast (2DPC) MRA

____ b. 2D time of flight (2DTOF) MRA

____ c. maximum intensity projection (MIP)

____ d. 3D time of flight (3DTOF) MRA

42. _____ is a technique that collects data continuously throuth the cardiac cycle.

____ a. Cine

____ b. MIP

____ c. EPI

____ d. MRA

43. Which of the following sequences best demonstrate the Circle of Willis?

____ a. 2DTOF

____ b. 3DTOF

____ c. 2DPC

____ d. 3DPC

44. Which of the following sequences best demonstrate the carotid arteries?

____ a. 2DTOF

____ b. 3DTOF

____ c. 2DPC

____ d. 3DPC

45. Cine is performed during a _____ pulse sequence.
    ___ a. spin density
    ___ b. gradient echo
    ___ c. TOF
    ___ d. IR

46. Which of the following techniques is the fastest of the high speed MR techniques?
    ___ a. TOF
    ___ b. MIP
    ___ c. EPI
    ___ d. CINE

47. Laminar flow at the center of the lumen of a vessel is _____ than at the wall of the vessel.
    ___ a. slower
    ___ b. faster
    ___ c. the same as
    ___ d. none of the above

48. _____ is flow at different velocities that fluctuate randomly. The velocity difference across the vessel changes erratically.
    ___ a. laminar flow
    ___ b. vortex flow
    ___ c. turbulent flow
    ___ d. none of the above

49. TOF effects depend on which of the following?
    ___ a. velocity of flow
    ___ b. echo time
    ___ c. slice thickness
    ___ d. all of the above

50. As the velocity of flow decreases, a higher proportion of flowing nuclei are present in a slice for both the 90° and the 180° RF pulses. Therefore, as the velocity of flow de-

creases, the TOF effect decreases. What is the name of this effect?

_____ a. low velocity signal loss

_____ b. array processing

_____ c. TOF

_____ d. flow-related enhancement

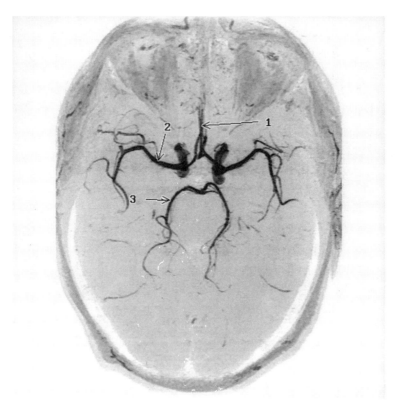

Figure 33

51. Identify structure 1 in Figure 33.

_____ a. carotid artery

_____ b. middle cerebral artery

_____ c. anterior cerebral artery

_____ d. posterior cerebral artery

52. Identify structure 2 in Figure 33.
    ___ a. right cerebral artery
    ___ b. left cerebral artery
    ___ c. middle cerebral artery
    ___ d. carotid bulb

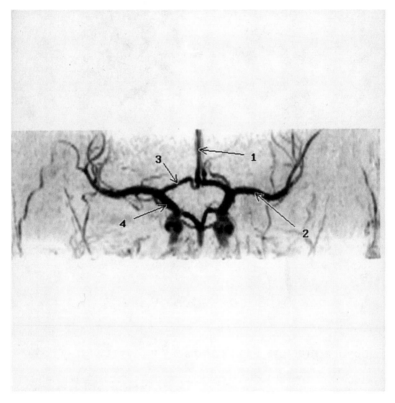

Figure 34

53. Identify structure 2 in Figure 34.
    ___ a. anterior cerebral artery
    ___ b. middle cerebral artery
    ___ c. carotid artery
    ___ d. anterior communicating artery

54. Identify structure 3 in Figure 34.
    ____ a. anterior cerebral artery
    ____ b. middle cerebral artery
    ____ c. anterior communicating artery
    ____ d. posterior communicating artery

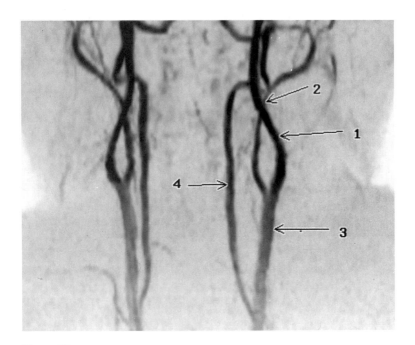

Figure 35

55. Identify structure 1 in Figure 35.
    ____ a. internal carotid artery
    ____ b. external carotid artery
    ____ c. siphon
    ____ d. vertebral artery

56. Identify structure 3 in Figure 35.
    ____ a. vertebral artery
    ____ b. common carotid artery
    ____ c. internal carotid artery
    ____ d. external carotid artery

57. Identify structure 4 in Figure 35.

_____ a. carotid artery

_____ b. vertebral artery

_____ c. middle carotid artery

_____ d. none of the above

58. On a sagittal projection, which structure is directly anterior to the uterus?

_____ a. cervix

_____ b. pubic symphysis

_____ c. ovary

_____ d. bladder

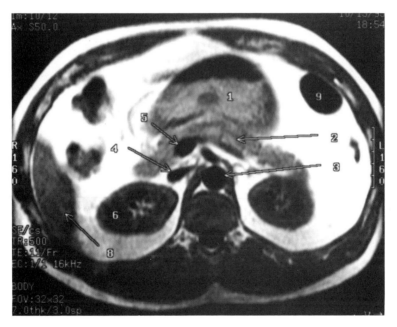

Figure 36

59. Identify structure 1 in Figure 36.

_____ a. bladder

_____ b. uterus

_____ c. stomach

_____ d. bowel

60. Identify structure 2 in Figure 36.

    _____ a. renal artery

    _____ b. pancreas

    _____ c. spleen

    _____ d. bowel

61. Identify structure 3 in Figure 36.

    _____ a. aorta

    _____ b. vena cava

    _____ c. splenic vein

    _____ d. portal vein

62. Identify structure 4 in Figure 36.

    _____ a. inferior vena cava

    _____ b. portal vein

    _____ c. superior mesenteric vein

    _____ d. splenic vein

63. Identify structure 9 in Figure 36.

    _____ a. stomach

    _____ b. bowel

    _____ c. kidney

    _____ d. aorta

64. Identify structure 8 in Figure 36.

    _____ a. stomach

    _____ b. spleen

    _____ c. liver

    _____ d. none of the above

65. In order to display a deep vein thrombosis in the femoral area, presaturation pulses should be placed in which direction?

    _____ a. superiorly

    _____ b. anteriorly

    _____ c. posteriorly

    _____ d. inferiorly

66. In order to display the carotid arteries, without the surrounding veins, select the location of the presaturation pulse.

____ a. superiorly
____ b. inferiorly
____ c. posteriorly
____ d. right to left

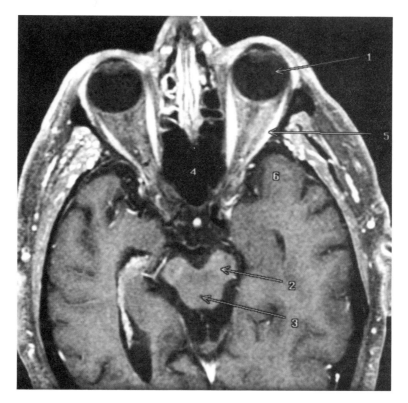

Figure 37

67. Which of the following is the technique employed to visualize the orbit in Figure 37?

____ a. gradient echo
____ b. spin echo
____ c. EPI
____ d. inversion recovery

68. Identify structure 4 in Figure 37.
    ___ a. sphenoid sinus
    ___ b. ethmoid sinus
    ___ c. superior sagittal sinus
    ___ d. insula

69. _____ is known as a rapidly developing tumor of the kidney that usually occurs in children.
    ___ a. Whipple's disease
    ___ b. Wilson's disease
    ___ c. Wilm's tumor
    ___ d. Renal sarcoidosis

70. The principal route of venous drainage is through a system of cerebral veins that empty into which of the following?
    ___ a. cavernous sinus
    ___ b. basal vein
    ___ c. jugular vein
    ___ d. vein of Galen

71. The pulse sequence interval from the 90° RF pulse to the collection of the MR signal is termed what?
    ___ a. TR
    ___ b. TE
    ___ c. tau
    ___ d. TI

72. The IR pulse sequence interval from the initial 180° RF pulse, used to flip the net magnetization into the negative "z" plane, to the 90° RF pulse is termed _____.
    ___ a. TR
    ___ b. TE
    ___ c. tau
    ___ d. TI

73. Which of the pulse sequences listed uses an initial RF pulse of less than 90°?
    1. fast GRE
    2. GRE
    3. 3DFT GRE

    ___ a. 1 only
    ___ b. 1 and 2 only
    ___ c. 2 and 3 only
    ___ d. 1, 2, and 3

74. In IR pulse sequences the "null point" is essential for which of the following?
    1. To find the area where the net magnetization intersects the transverse plane.
    2. To determine what TI time causes the suppression of a tissue.
    3. To determine when 69% of the tissues T1 relaxation has occurred.

    ___ a. 1 only
    ___ b. 1 and 2 only
    ___ c. 2 and 3 only
    ___ d. 1, 2, and 3

75. Which of the pulse sequences below is capable of producing true T2-weighted images?
    1. GRE
    2. conventional double SE
    3. FSE

    ___ a. 2 only
    ___ b. 1 and 2 only
    ___ c. 2 and 3 only
    ___ d. 1, 2, and 3

76. Magnetic susceptibility effects are seen most prominent in which pulse sequence below?
    ____ a. IR
    ____ b. CSE
    ____ c. GRE
    ____ d. FSE

77. What type of flip angles do GRE pulse sequences use?
    ____ a. 90°
    ____ b. less than 90°
    ____ c. more than 90°
    ____ d. the Ernst angle

78. In a conventional double SE pulse sequence using a long TR, what is the type of contrast usually acquired?
    ____ a. 1st echo — T2-weighted
         2nd echo — T2-weighted
    ____ b. 1st echo — T1-weighted
         2nd echo — PD-weighted
    ____ c. 1st echo — PD-weighted
         2nd echo — T2*-weighted
    ____ d. 1st echo — PD-weighted
         2nd echo — T2-weighted

79. In a 3DFT pulse sequence, increasing the number of slices from 32 to 64 slices causes what result?
    1. an increase in SNR
    2. an increase in scan time
    3. an increase in slice thickness

    ____ a. 1 only
    ____ b. 1 and 2 only
    ____ c. 2 and 3 only
    ____ d. 1, 2, and 3

80. In FSE pulse sequences what parameter is most responsible for image contrast?

    ____ a. TR

    ____ b. ETE

    ____ c. ETL

    ____ d. flip angle

81. What process must occur in spin echo imaging to rephase that portion of the net magnetization that has been dephased over time after the application of the initial 90° RF pulse?

    1. gradient reversal

    2. 180° RF pulse

    3. 90° RF pulse

    ____ a. 1 only

    ____ b. 2 only

    ____ c. 1 and 2 only

    ____ d. 1, 2, and 3

82. If fractional averaging or partial (half) Fourier imaging is used in a 2D sequence, approximately what percentage of SNR is reduced compared with a conventional one NEX 2D sequence?

    ____ a. 30

    ____ b. 41

    ____ c. 50

    ____ d. 70

83. When only part of the signal is read by the frequency-encoding gradient, it is called _____.

    1. partial averaging

    2. zero filling

    3. partial or fractional echo

    ____ a. 1 only

    ____ b. 3 only

    ____ c. 1 and 3 only

    ____ d. 1, 2, and 3

84. Which of the statements below are true regarding partial or fractional averaging?
    1. As long as at least half of the lines of k-space are filled, enough data exists to produce an image.
    2. Scan time is not affected when performing partial averaging.
    3. This is also called zero filling.

    ____ a. 1 only
    ____ b. 3 only
    ____ c. 1 and 3 only
    ____ d. 1, 2, and 3

85. A mathematical technique that allows an MR signal to be decomposed into a sum of sine waves of different frequencies, phases, and amplitudes is called

    _____.

    ____ a. conjugate synthesis
    ____ b. Fourier transform
    ____ c. MIP
    ____ d. sinc function

86. The center frequency of the RF pulse determines the location of the slice, whereas the RF bandwidth determines

    _____.

    ____ a. signal amplitude
    ____ b. phase direction
    ____ c. slice thickness
    ____ d. echo time

87. Which of the statements below is true of partial or fractional echo imaging?
    1. The echo no longer has to be centered on the middle of the frequency encoding gradient.
    2. The TE can be reduced because the peak of the echo can occur closer to the RF pulse.
    3. The sampling window is shifted during readout so that only the peak and the dephasing part of the echo are sampled.

    ___ a. 1 only
    ___ b. 2 only
    ___ c. 1 and 2 only
    ___ d. 1, 2, and 3

88. If the RF bandwidth remains constant, how can slice thickness be changed?
    1. By changing the slope of the slice-select gradient.
    2. By changing the rise time of the slice-select gradient.
    3. By changing the strength of the slice-select gradient.

    ___ a. 1 only
    ___ b. 2 only
    ___ c. 1 and 3 only
    ___ d. 2 and 3 only

89. TOF MRA, 2DFT or 3DFT is based on the use of which of the following parameters?
    1. gradient moment nulling
    2. moderate to large flip angles ($30°$ to $60°$)
    3. very short TE times (less than 5-7 msec)

    ___ a. 1 only
    ___ b. 1 and 3 only
    ___ c. 1 and 2 only
    ___ d. 1, 2, and 3

90. A GRE pulse sequence that uses bipolar flow-encoding gradients along one or more axes is indicative of which type of pulse sequence?
    ___ a. GRE in the steady state
    ___ b. phase contrast MRA
    ___ c. rephase/dephase MRA
    ___ d. fast GRE

91. Maximum enhancement of flow occurs when the vessel is _____ in relation to the plane of imaging.
    ___ a. adjacent
    ___ b. parallel
    ___ c. perpendicular
    ___ d. against

92. What is the unit of measurement for VENC, velocity encoding?
    ___ a. cm/sec^2
    ___ b. $cm^2/msec$
    ___ c. cm/sec
    ___ d. cm/msec

93. Spins moving with constant velocity experience a phase shift that is proportional to which of the following?
    1. flow velocity
    2. amplitude of the bipolar gradient
    3. time interval between the gradient lobes

    ___ a. 1 only
    ___ b. 3 only
    ___ c. 1 and 3 only
    ___ d. 1, 2, and 3

94. Which pulse sequence is most useful for imaging relatively rapid flow in vessels passing perpendicular to the plane of imaging?
    ___ a. TOF MRA
    ___ b. 2D PC MRA
    ___ c. rephase/dephase MRA
    ___ d. 3D PC MRA

95. T1-weighted SE images are acquired using the following parameters?
    ___ a. short TR and short TE
    ___ b. long TR and long TE
    ___ c. short TR and long TE
    ___ d. long TR and short TE

96. K-space refers to
    ___ a. storage of extra data sets
    ___ b. storage of processed data
    ___ c. storage of raw data
    ___ d. storage of phase encoding projection

97. The contrast and SNR information is located _____ of k-space.
    ___ a. on the outer lines
    ___ b. on the central lines
    ___ c. on the center line
    ___ d. on the bottom half

98. Which parameter can be adjusted to shorten scan time without affecting image contrast?
    ___ a. flip angle
    ___ b. matrix size
    ___ c. gradient reversal
    ___ d. fractional echo

99. A SE image created using a long TR and a short TE produces _____ contrast.

____ a. T1-weighted
____ b. T2-weighted
____ c. T2*-weighted
____ d. PD-weighted

100. How does increasing the matrix in the frequency direction from 256 to 512 affect image acquisition?

1. It will increase the scan time two fold.
2. It will increase resolution.
3. It will limit frequency aliasing.

____ a. 1 only
____ b. 2 only
____ c. 2 and 3 only
____ d. 1 and 3 only

101. Which of the following are important in determining the phase-encoding direction of an image acquisition?

1. Phase encode perpendicular to the direction of flow or motion when possible.
2. Phase encode on the short axis of the patient.
3. Phase encode in the direction where the most signal is needed.

____ a. 1 only
____ b. 2 only
____ c. 1 and 2 only
____ d. 1, 2, and 3

102. In CSE multislice imaging what happens to the maximum number of slices allowed when TR increases?
    ___ a. no effect when increasing TR
    ___ b. the number of slices increases at a ratio of TR/TE
    ___ c. the number of slices decreases by a factor of the TR
    ___ d. the number of slices decreases at a ratio of TR/TE

103. Reducing the NEX _____ SNR.
    ___ a. increases
    ___ b. reduces
    ___ c. no effect on
    ___ d. doubles

104. Increasing the number of phase encode steps while maintaining FOV causes what effect?
    1. an increase in scan time
    2. an increase in spatial resolution
    3. an increase in coverage

    ___ a. 1 only
    ___ b. 1 and 2 only
    ___ c. 2 and 3 only
    ___ d. 1, 2, and 3

105. What imaging parameter is most responsible for contrast when acquiring IR pulse sequences?
    ___ a. TR
    ___ b. TE
    ___ c. TI
    ___ d. flip angle

106. STIR sequences are useful in suppressing the signal from which of the following tissues?
    1. fat
    2. water
    3. gadolinium enhancing lesion

    ___ a. 1 only
    ___ b. 2 only
    ___ c. 1 and 3 only
    ___ d. 1, 2, and 3

107. What result would be expected in a SE pulse sequence if the TE is reduced?

    ___ a. increase in T2-weighting
    ___ b. decrease in scan time
    ___ c. increase in PD-weighting
    ___ d. decrease in T1-weighting

108. Pixel size is equal to which of the following?

    ___ a. matrix size/FOV
    ___ b. FOV/matrix size
    ___ c. frequency encoding/matrix
    ___ d. phase encoding/matrix

109. What relationship does SNR have to voxel volume?

    ___ a. SNR is inversely proportional to voxel volume
    ___ b. SNR is proportional to voxel volume
    ___ c. Doubling the voxel volume halves the SNR
    ___ d. Doubling the voxel volume changes SNR by the square root of the change

110. Which pulse sequence converts only a portion of the longitudinal magnetization into transverse magnetization?

    ___ a. IR
    ___ b. GRE
    ___ c. partial saturation
    ___ d. inversion SE

111. Increasing the number of frequency encoding steps will:
  1. increase scan time
  2. increase spatial resolution
  3. decrease frequency aliasing

  ___ a. 1 only
  ___ b. 2 only
  ___ c. 2 and 3 only
  ___ d. 1, 2, and 3

112. What controls the amount of transverse magnetization that is allowed to decay before an echo is collected?

  ___ a. TR
  ___ b. flip angle
  ___ c. TE
  ___ d. T2

113. What describes the number of times data is collected with the same amplitude of phase encoding gradient called?
  1. number of averages
  2. number of excitations
  3. number of acquisitions

  ___ a. 1 only
  ___ b. 1 and 2 only
  ___ c. 2 only
  ___ d. 1, 2, and 3

114. The presence of random noise causes the doubling the NEX to increase SNR by _____.

  ___ a. one-fourth
  ___ b. $\sqrt{2}$
  ___ c. half
  ___ d. double

115. What change in receive bandwidth would need to be made to collect less noise in a sample?
    ____ a. bandwidth should be decreased
    ____ b. bandwidth should be increased
    ____ c. bandwidth will not affect noise collection
    ____ d. bandwidth causes increased signal to be collected

116. What determines the number of pixels in the FOV?
    ____ a. slice thickness
    ____ b. matrix size
    ____ c. voxel size
    ____ d. resolution

117. Which of the following parameters, if reduced, and providing all other parameters remain the same, causes partial voluming to be reduced?
    1. pixel size
    2. field of view
    3. slice thickness

    ____ a. 1 only
    ____ b. 2 only
    ____ c. 1 and 3 only
    ____ d. 1, 2, and 3

118. Doubling the FOV doubles the voxel volume along both axes and has what effect on SNR?
    ____ a. SNR halves
    ____ b. SNR doubles
    ____ c. SNR quadruples
    ____ d. SNR remains the same

119. When acquiring CSE multislice images the number of slices allowed, if the TE decreases from 50 msec to 35 msec:

    ____ a. increases

    ____ b. decreases

    ____ c. doubles

    ____ d. is not affected by TE time

120. Sampling alternate phase encode lines in k-space while leaving the maximum and minimum amplitudes of the phase-encoding gradient unchanged causes what result?

    ____ a. gradient spoiling

    ____ b. rectangular FOV

    ____ c. partial NEX

    ____ d. half-Fourier imaging

121. Which of the technologist choices below is not recommended with a patient who is likely to move during the scan?

    ____ a. use the shortest TR possible

    ____ b. reduce the NEX to a minimum

    ____ c. use the smallest matrix size possible

    ____ d. use gradient echo sequences to reduce scan time

122. Which factor is SNR proportional to?

    1. 1/ receive bandwidth

    2. 1/ number of frequency encodings

    3. 1/ number of phase encodings

    ____ a. 1 only

    ____ b. 1 and 2

    ____ c. 2 only

    ____ d. 1, 2, and 3

123. How is it possible to obtain equal spatial resolution in every plane and at every angle of obliquity?
    1. use symmetrical voxels
    2. use isotropic voxels
    3. use anisotropic voxels

    ___ a. 1 only
    ___ b. 2 only
    ___ c. 1 and 3 only
    ___ d. 1 and 2 only

124. How can the SNR of an entire FOV increase?
    ___ a. decrease the flip angle
    ___ b. volume imaging
    ___ c. conjugate synthesis
    ___ d. broad receive bandwidth

125. In FSE imaging, the distance between successive echoes is called:
    ___ a. echo train length (ETL)
    ___ b. effective echo
    ___ c. echo train spacing (ETS)
    ___ d. echo train time

126. If phase encode steps, slice thickness, and flip angle are all increased, what combined result would you expect regarding image quality?
    ___ a. contrast increases
    ___ b. SNR increases
    ___ c. spatial resolution increases
    ___ d. scan time decreases

127. If the FOV, TR, and number of slices in volume imaging are reduced, what combined result would you expect regarding image quality?
    ___ a. contrast increases
    ___ b. SNR decreases
    ___ c. spatial resolution increases
    ___ d. scan time increases

128. IF TR is increased, TE is decreased, and receive bandwidth is decreased, what combined result would be expected?
    ___ a. contrast increases
    ___ b. SNR increases
    ___ c. spatial resolution increases
    ___ d. scan time decreases

129. If the slice thickness is decreased, FOV is decreased, and matrix is increased what combined result would be expected?
    ___ a. contrast increases
    ___ b. SNR increases
    ___ c. spatial resolution increases
    ___ d. scan time decreases

130. If a matrix size of 256 x 256 is used with an FOV of 16 x 16 cm, what is the resolution or size of the pixel?
    ___ a. .0625 x .0625 mm
    ___ b. .625 x .625 mm
    ___ c. 1.6 x 1.6 mm
    ___ d. 16 x 16 mm

131. Images acquired using a long TE time may result in which of the following image quality results?

    1. lower SNR
    2. higher image graininess
    3. lower T2 contrast

    ____ a. 1 only
    ____ b. 2 only
    ____ c. 1 and 2 only
    ____ d. 1, 2, and 3

132. Each slice of an image consists of a series of volume elements called _____.

    ____ a. vectors
    ____ b. pixels
    ____ c. voxels
    ____ d. protons

133. What law states that a changing magnetic field generates a voltage and current in a conductor?

    ____ a. Ohm's law
    ____ b. Faraday's law
    ____ c. Tesla's law
    ____ d. Gauss's law

134. MR systems are required to be homogeneous to be effective as a clinical device. What device assures homogeneity of the static magnetic field?

    1. magnetic shields
    2. shim coils
    3. RF shields

    ____ a. 1 only
    ____ b. 2 only
    ____ c. 1 and 2 only
    ____ d. 1, 2, and 3

135. What is the most common type of magnet designed for clinical MR imaging?
    ___ a. permanent
    ___ b. air-core resistive
    ___ c. iron-core resistive
    ___ d. superconductive

136. Which magnet type is capable of producing magnetic fields greater than 1 T?
    1. permanent
    2. resistive
    3. superconductive

    ___ a. 2 and 3 only
    ___ b. 3 only
    ___ c. 2 only
    ___ d. 1, 2, and 3

137. Which of the magnet types require the use of solenoidal coils to transmit the RF energy necessary to excite the atoms?
    1. permanent
    2. iron-core resistive
    3. air-core resistive

    ___ a. 1 only
    ___ b. 1 and 2 only
    ___ c. 1 and 3 only
    ___ d. 1, 2, and 3

138. Increasing the size of the receive coil will increase the available FOV and will _____ SNR.
    ___ a. increase
    ___ b. decrease
    ___ c. double
    ___ d. doubles

139. The energy transmitted at the resonant frequency of hydrogen in the form of a short intense burst is known as

_____.

____ a. precessional frequency
____ b. RF pulse
____ c. center frequency
____ d. bandwidth

140. To avoid coupling, the RF pulse must be applied _____ to the main magnetic field B_0.

____ a. parallel
____ b. perpendicular
____ c. adjacent
____ d. tangential

141. What component is responsible for supplying power to the gradient coils?

____ a. RF transmit coil
____ b. operating computer
____ c. gradient amplifier
____ d. RF amplifier

142. Which substance when placed in a strong magnetic field shows strong attraction to it, aligns with it, and retains its absorbed magnetization?

____ a. gyromagnetic
____ b. paramagnetic
____ c. ferromagnetic
____ d. diamagnetic

143. What term describes the relationship between the electron configuration of an atom and the ability of external magnetic fields to affect the nucleus of that atom?

____ a. magnetism
____ b. magnetic susceptibility
____ c. chemical shift
____ d. pseudomagnetism

144. The secondary oscillating magnetic field (B_1) formed as a result of passing current through a loop of wire is called?
_____ a. gradient magnetic field
_____ b. magnetic susceptibility
_____ c. RF pulse
_____ d. static magnetic field

145. The RF pulse transmitted to excite a slice must contain a range of frequencies to match the difference in precessional frequency between two points. What is this range called?
_____ a. RF pulse
_____ b. transmit bandwidth
_____ c. receive bandwidth
_____ d. precessional frequency

146. What determines the size of the gap between slices?
_____ a. transmit bandwidth and the slice thickness
_____ b. gradient slope and the thickness of the slice
_____ c. RF pulse and the slice thickness
_____ d. gradient slope and the receive bandwidth

147. A situation in which the action of three or more unequally spaced RF pulses produce additional echoes is called _____.
_____ a. rephased echo
_____ b. stimulated echo
_____ c. simulated echo
_____ d. spin echo

148. The wobbling movement of the nucleus as it spins on its own axis is called _____.
_____ a. spin warp
_____ b. resonance
_____ c. pseudofrequency
_____ d. precession

149. What is the precessional frequency necessary to excite hydrogen atoms exposed to a 1.9 T magnetic field?

___ a. 63.9 mHz

___ b. 80.9 mHz

___ c. 85.5 mHz

___ d. 86.0 mHz

150. The length of time it takes the net magnetization vector to return to equilibrium after RF excitation is called

_____.

___ a. T1 relaxation

___ b. T2 relaxation

___ c. longitudinal relaxation

___ d. relaxation time

151. The strength and direction of a tissue's combined response to the static magnetic fields is called

_____.

___ a. net magnetism

___ b. transverse magnetism

___ c. net magnetic vector

___ d. magnetic susceptibility

152. Energy transmitted at the precessional frequency of hydrogen in a magnetic field causes _____ to occur.

___ a. precession

___ b. resonance

___ c. net magnetization

___ d. coupling

153. What does the amplitude and the duration of the RF pulse determine?

___ a. net magnetization

___ b. precessional frequency

___ c. flip angle

___ d. net magnetic vector

154. As the net magnetic vector precesses at the Larmor frequency in the transverse plane, _____ is
induced into the receive coil.
      ____ a. signal
      ____ b. coupling
      ____ c. resonance
      ____ d. voltage

155. As the magnitude of transverse magnetization decreases,
so does the magnitude of the voltage induced in the receiver coil. What is this decrease called?
      ____ a. longitudinal relaxation
      ____ b. FID
      ____ c. MR signal
      ____ d. relaxation

156. The relaxation resulting from the loss of transverse magnetization due to interactions between the magnetic fields
of adjacent nuclei is called _____.
      ____ a. relaxation time
      ____ b. T1 relaxation
      ____ c. T2 relaxation
      ____ d. FID

157. Reducing the amplitude of the readout gradient while prolonging its length results in an echo that is "spread out"
in time. What is this procedure called?
      1. extended sampling time
      2. variable bandwidth
      3. fractional echo

      ____ a. 1 only
      ____ b. 2 only
      ____ c. 3 only
      ____ d. 1 and 2 only

158. Gradient lobes that are added before signal readout to compensate in advance for motion-induced dephasing at the time of the echo is termed _____.
     1. gradient moment nulling
     2. gradient motion rephasing
     3. flow compensation

     ____ a. 1 only
     ____ b. 2 only
     ____ c. 1 and 3 only
     ____ d. 1, 2, and 3

159. What is the scan time of the following pulse sequence?

TR	3000 msec	ETS	20 msec
FA	90°	Matrix	256 x 256
ETE	90 msec	NEX	4
ETL	16	FOV	24 x 24 cm

     ____ a. 3.2 minutes
     ____ b. 6.4 minutes
     ____ c. 16 minutes
     ____ d. 51 minutes

160. Which of the components below can be directly measured with MRI?
     1. longitudinal magnetization
     2. transverse magnetization
     3. spin density

     ____ a. 1 only
     ____ b. 2 only
     ____ c. 2 and 3 only
     ____ d. 1, 2, and 3

161. Any measurement based on the image signal intensity is actually the average determination from which part of the voxel?
    ____ a. signal averaged across adjacent voxels
    ____ b. signal averaged from the entire voxel
    ____ c. signal averaged from the end value of voxels
    ____ d. signal averaged from surrounding voxels

162. The x-gradient superimposes a linearly distorted magnetic field that varies the magnetic field strength in the _____ direction in reference to the patient.
    ____ a. anterior to posterior
    ____ b. inferior to superior
    ____ c. left to right
    ____ d. caudal to cephalic

163. The representation of the MR signal converted to amplitude vs. time is called _____.
    ____ a. Fourier transformation
    ____ b. time domain
    ____ c. processed domain
    ____ d. frequency domain

164. Changes in precession angle or phase that protons undergo when they move within a magnetic field gradient is termed _____.
    ____ a. flow enhancement
    ____ b. spin phase effects
    ____ c. acceleration
    ____ d. phase dispersions

165. A process that is accomplished by using three distinct steps in which each encodes a different spatial axis of a slice is called _____.
    1. 2DFT imaging
    2. 3DFT imaging
    3. Spatial encoding

    ____ a. 1 only
    ____ b. 1 and 3 only
    ____ c. 3 only
    ____ d. 2 and 3 only

166. _____ creates a one-to-one correspondence between the frequency of the returned signal and the source's position along the readout direction.

    ____ a. frequency-encoding gradient
    ____ b. receive bandwidth
    ____ c. Fourier transformation
    ____ d. receive coil

167. Which of the fat suppression techniques below is produced using IR pulse sequences?

    ____ a. phase evolution, Dixon method
    ____ b. frequency-selective excitation "fat sat"
    ____ c. T1-dependent suppression
    ____ d. selective water excitation, slice-selective gradient reversal

168. What is the amount of signal from flow recorded as a result of entry phenomenon proportional to?

    ____ a. the pulse sequence
    ____ b. slice thickness and repetition time
    ____ c. echo time
    ____ d. tissue's relaxation time

169. What is the process called in which laminar flow is back in phase after the application of the 90° RF pulse and two

symmetrical echoes are collected subsequent to equally spaced 180° RF pulses?

____ a. rephasing

____ b. transverse remagnetization

____ c. even echo rephasing

____ d. double echo rephasing

170. The ambiguous assignment of frequencies to the MR signal can cause _____ artifact.

____ a. motion

____ b. aliasing

____ c. inhomogeneous brightness

____ d. ghosting

171. What is the cause of the chemical shift artifact phenomenon?

____ a. the electron cloud of fat and water

____ b. the nuclear configuration of fat and water

____ c. the proton concentration of fat and water

____ d. the chemical imbalance of fat and water

172. What is the actual chemical shift of fat and water exposed to a 1.5 T magnetic field?

____ a. 63 Hz

____ b. 63 mHz

____ c. 224 Hz

____ d. 224 mHz

173. An artifact that results because the first peak of the sine wave adjacent to the high-contrast interface always over-shoots the ideal intensity line to a greater degree than subsequent peaks is called _____.

    1. truncation artifact
    2. chemical shift artifact
    3. Gibb's artifact

    ___ a. 1 only
    ___ b. 3 only
    ___ c. 1 and 2 only
    ___ d. 1 and 3 only

174. The B1 magnetic field is produced by which coil?

    ___ a. main magnet
    ___ b. gradient
    ___ c. RF transmit
    ___ d. shim

175. What effect do paramagnetic substances have on tissue relaxation?

    1. T1 relaxation is shortened.
    2. T2 relaxation is shortened.
    3. T2 relaxation is lengthened.

    ___ a. 1 only
    ___ b. 3 only
    ___ c. 1 and 2 only
    ___ d. 1 and 3 only

Answers

1. (d) Not only is it important to identify magnetic materials within the patient that may cause injury or burn, it is also important to acquire pertinent history concerning the patient. Symptoms, onset of pain, and previous surgery are all valuable information to the radiologist. Explaining the procedure helps to develop rapport with the patient and allay their fears. **SH**

2. (d) Any person who enters the scan room is exposed to the static magnetic field and should therefore, be asked basic screening questions. **SH**

3. (c) Intra-occular ferrous fragments may be easily seen on plain film radiographs. **POTT**

4. (d) Studies have shown that iron, nickel, and cobalt are all ferromagnetic materials. **WO**

5. (d) Within six weeks after surgery, scar tissue has formed around a thoracic aneurysm clip, making it safe to scan. Nonferrous intracranial aneurysm clips are not attracted to the magnetic field. **SH**

6. (b) Both the cochlear implants and the Duraphase penile implants have shown ferrous qualities. **SH**

7. (b) "Although MRI is not presently considered hazardous to the fetus, the safety has not yet been established. Since there is a high spontaneous abortion rate in the general population during the first trimester of pregnancy, particular care should be exercised." **SH**

8. (d) The static magnetic field may interfere with implants that are electrically, magnetically, or mechanically activated. Therefore, patients that have neurostimulators, bone growth stimulators, or implanted drug infusion pumps are contraindicated for scanning. **ST**

9. (d) A ferrous piece of shrapnel may torque in the magnetic field and tear the popliteal vessel located in the posterior area of the knee. Fatio eyelid springs are made from a ferromagnetic form of stainless steel that could injure the eye. Epicardial leads that

are left in the chest after surgery induce current and cause severe burns. **SH**

10. (c) In order to prevent the pediatric patient from vomiting and ingesting emesis into the lungs, the patient should be without food or water (NPO) for at least 4 hours before sedation. **POTT**

11. (a) The most commonly reported reaction to contrast is a mild transitory headache. **SH**

12. (a) Epinephrine is usually the drug of choice that is administered during severe bronchospasm. **SC**

13. (d) All patients should be visually and verbally monitored during their scan. **SH**

14. (d) Increasing the oxygen to a level of 10 could cause a COPD patient to stop breathing. Stopping the scan and checking with the nurse who is in charge of the patient, and who is familiar with that patient's condition is very important. **POTT**

15. (d) Normal oxygen levels should be around 95%-100%. **POTT**

16. (a) The normal pulse rate is around 60-100 beats per minute. **POTT**

17. (a) According to the FDA, a severe reaction to MR contrast is described as life threatening or permanently disabling. **SH**

18. (d) It is adviseable to place monitoring devices approximately 8 feet from the bore of a 1.5T magnet. **ST**

19. (d) Both permanent and resistive magnets have a range of about 0.3T. Low field superconductive magnets are generally around 0.5T. A high field superconductive magnet has a field strength of above 1T. The higher the field strength, the stronger the attraction to projectiles. **BU**

20. (d) Education of the personnel and patients is the most important aspect of providing a safe MR environment. **POTT**

21. (c) The fringe magnetic field may be reduced passively by using large amounts of steel in the walls of the magnet room. **BU**

22. (a) The wires on the ECG monitor and surface cable have potential to induce current and cause patient

burns. The pulse oximeter is made from fiberoptics which do not induce current. **SH**

23. (a) The environmental temperature should be around 65-75° F.

24. (b) In order to prevent extraneous RF from entering the scan room, copper is placed around the scan room. This is called a Faraday cage. **BU**

25. (b) The exclusion zone is at the 5G level. **POTT**

26. (d) All of the choices have ferromagnetic properties. **SH**

27. (a) The humidity in a scan environment should be around 50-70.

28. (c) A quench is the sudden, rapid boil off of cryogens. **POTT**

29. (d) In a quench, the oxygen in the room may be quickly replaced by helium. This gaseous helium is extrmely cold and may cause frostbite and asphyxiation. **SH**

30. (b) During a quench, helium quickly replaces the oxygen and forms a cloud, with a small amount of oxygen close to the floor. **SH**

31. (d) Patients with sickle cell anemia may progress to sickle cell crisis following an injection of gadolinium. Pregnant patients and nursing mothers are also contraindicated. "Contrast has been shown to cross the placenta and appear in the fetal bladder shortly after injection in the mother. Contrast is then excreted from the fetal bladder into the amniotic fluid which is later swallowed by the fetus. This cycle occurs many times." At the present, there is no data to assess the rate of clearance from the amniotic cycle. Contrast has been shown to be excreted in breast milk. Nursing mothers are instructed to express their breasts and not to nurse their children for 36-48 hours post contrast. **MA,OM,PR,SH**

32. (c) Electrically conductive surface coil cables should be kept away form the outside bore of the magnet, away from patient's skin and positioned to avoid looping or "crosspoints." **SH**

33. (d) All of the choices are correct. Contrast agents should be placed away from direct sunlight. Freezing may cause cracks in the container. Because there are no preservatives in contrast agents, they should only be drawn up minutes before injecting. **OM,PR,MA**

34. (c) Cables that are crossed or looped may form a conductor, which could cause patient burns. **SH**

35. (c) The farther the coil is from the patient, the lower the SNR. **BU**

36. (d) If a patient's arm touches the magnet, patient burn, detuning of the magnet, and degraded images due to increased RG disposition may (all) occur.

37. (a) The respiratory belt has no wires which could cause a conductive loop. **SH**

38. (c) During an MRI scan, the patient is exposed to three forms of electromagnetic radiation: from the static magnetic field, the gradient field, and the RF electromagnetic fields. **ST**

39. (c) The current FDA limit is magnetic fields up to 2T. **ST**

40. (d) All of the answers are synonymous. **SH**

41. (a) The magnetic field is measured in tesla (T) at isocenter and gauss (G) outside of the magnet. **POTT**

42. (a) FDA has determined the SAR limit to .4W per Kg. **ST**

43. (b) SAR is the term applied to RF absorbtion by the body during scanning. **ST**

44. (a) RF fields should not cause the body core temperature to rise more than 1° C. **ST**

45. (c) Studies show that there is more body heating on the outside surface of the body core than in the middle. **SH**

46. (a) The photoplethysmograph records the patient's heart rate. **SH**

47. (b) The blood pressure cuff is called a sphygmomaneter. **SH**

48. (c) Organs that have reduced capacity for heat dissipation are the testes and the eye, which makes them

particularily sensitive to elevated temperature from excessive RF exposure. **SH**

49. (b) The capnometer or pulse oximeter is considered to be a standard practice for monitoring sedated or anesthetized patients. **SH**

50. (a) The "missile effect" poses the largest problem when dealing with ferromagnetic materials in a static magnetic field. **ST**

51. (a) The linear gradient alters the magnetic field by 1G per cm. **POTT**

52. (c) Gadolinium is bound to a chelate to decrease the amount of toxicity in the body. **SH**

53. (a) The gradient magnetic field is measured in G per cm or mTm. **ST**

54. (b) The coronal plane divides the head into anterior and posterior portions. **BU**

55. (a) The dura mater is the hard, exterior layer of meninges. **AP**

56. (d) Cisterns are the enlarged subarachnoid spaces. **AP**

57. (a) The superficial bulges on the surface of the cerbrum are called gyri. The dips or grooves are called sulci. **TA**

58. (a) Arrow 1 in Figure 1 is the temporal lobe. **AP**

    (Key to Figure 1: 1. Temporal lobe; 2. Parietal lobe; 3. Occipital lobe; 4. Frontal lobe.)

59. (a) The sylvian fissure in Figure 1 is located above the temporal lobe. **AP**

60. (c) The diencephalon is comprised of the epithalamus, thalamus, and hypothalamus. **AP**

61. (a) The tissue around the orbit is fatty in nature and appears bright on T1 sequences. **BU**

    (Key to Figure 2: 1. Cerebellum; 2. Internal auditory canal (IAC); 3. Occular bulb; 4. Maxillary sinus; 5. Intraorbital fat.)

62. (d) Arrow 2 in Figure 2 points to the 7th and 8th cranial nerves. A,B,and C are synonymous. **BU**

63. (b) The 7th cranial nerve is considered the facial nerve. **AP**

64. (d) The 8th cranial nerve affects hearing and balance. **AP**

65. (a) An acoustic neuroma is a benign tumor located in the 7th and 8th cranial nerves. It manifests itself in hearing loss, dizziness (vertigo) and/or ringing in the ears (tinnitus). **TA**

66. (a) Number 9 in Figure 3 denotes the anterior portion of the corpus callosum that is known the genu. **AP**

    (Key to Figure 3: 1. Cerebellum; 2. Second cervical vertebral body (C2); 3. Pons; 4. Medulla; 5. Thalamus; 6. Hypothalamus; 7. Pituitary gland; 8. Optic chiasm; 9. Genu of the corpus callosum; 10. Splenium of the corpus callosum; 11. Third ventricle; 12. Tentorium.)

67. (c) Number 3 in Figure 3 shows the pons, a rounded eminence on the ventral surface of the brainstem. It lies between the medulla and the cerebral peduncles.

68. (b) The medulla is located at the lower portion of the brainstem. (Number 4, Figure 3) **AP**

69. (b) The tentorium is a tent-like process of duramater between the cerebrum and the cerbellum. (Arrow 12 in Figure 3) **AP**

70. (d) The thalamus is a gray matter structure. (Structure 5 in Figure 3) **AP**

71. (d) Arrow 8 in Figure 3 points to the optic chiasm. **BU**

72. (a) Number 7 in Figure 3 is the pituitary gland. **BU**

73. (b) The pons is considered to be part of the brainstem. (Number 3 in Figure 3) **AP**

74. (d) Chiari malformation is a condition in which the inferior poles of the cerebrum protrude through the foramen magnum, creating intracranial pressure. **TA**

75. (d) In order to correctly image the pituitary gland, high resolution images are neccessary. One should employ a small FOV (about 16-18), thin slices (3 skip 1 mm or less) and a fine matrix (192-256) for best resolution. **BU**

76. (a) Bands of high and low signal intensity running parallel to tissue interface may often resemble a syrinx. This is particularily a problem in the cervical spine area. Enlarging the FOV or increasing the matrix provides better definition of this area. **ST**

77. (a) In order to visulize the internal auditory canal, high resolution images should be acquired in the axial and coronal planes. **BU**

78. (c) Sagittal and coronal planes best display the pituitary area. **BU**

79. (d) Hemorrhage displays high signal intensity on both T1- and T2-weighted images. **BU**

80. (c) Number 2 in Figure 4 is the ethmoid sinus. **BU**

(Key to Figure 4: 1. Frontal sinus; 2. Ethmoid sinus; 3. Sphenoid sinus; 4. Carotid siphon; 5. Cerebellar tonsil.)

81. (d) Number 3 in Figure 4 is the sphenoid sinus. **BU**

82. (a) Number 1 in Figure 4 is the frontal sinus. **BU**

83. (b) A gradient echo sequence is often helpful in identifying hemorrhage. **BU**

84. (d) IR sequences may help define gray/white matter structures in pediatric patients. **BU**

85. (a) The quadrature, head coil transmits and receives signal through two ports. **POTT**

86. (a) The putamen and globus pallidus make up the lentiform nucleus. **AP**

87. (d) Meningiomas are slow growing isointense tumors that originate from arachnoid tissue. **TA**

88. (b) Structure 1 in Figure 5 is the anterior cerebral artery. **MO**

(Key to Figure 5: 1. Genu of the corpus callosum; 2. Caudate nucleus; 3. Lentiform nucleus (Globus pallodus and putamen); 4. Internal capsule; 5. Middle cerebral artery; 6. White matter; 7. Gray matter.)

89. (a) Structue 2 in Figure 5 is the caudate nucleus. **MO**

90. (b) Structue 3 in Figure 5 is the globus pallidus. **MO**

91. (a) The internal capsule, marked 4 in Figure 5, is a white matter structure. **AP**

92. (c) Figure 5 was scanned in proton density (intermediate weighted) pulse sequence. **BU**

93. (c) Number 5 in Figure 5 points to the middle cerbral artery. **MO**

94. (a) The esophogas is located in closest proximity to the vertebrae on a sagittal cervical image. **MO**

95. (c) Lymph nodes are frequently isointense and the adjacent vessels are dark on T1 weighted images of the neck. **BU**

96. (c) The nasopharynx is the most superior portion of the pharynx. **MO**

97. (c) Sagittal T2-weighted images best demonstrate the amount of water or hydration in intervertebral discs. **BU**

98. (a) The sagittal plane best demonstrates spinal stenosis. **BU**

99. (b) Since the gradient echo sequence has no 180° refocusing pulse, it is most susceptible to inhomogeneities within the tissue. **BU**

100. (c) The lumbar area is least affected by CSF pulsatation artifacts. **BU**

101. (a) Structure 1 in Figure 6 is the cerebellar tonsil. **BU**
(Key to Figure 6: 1. Cerebellar tonsil; 2. Posterior arch of C1; 3. Spinous process; 4. Esophagus; 5. Trachea; 6. Vertebral body (C5); 7. Epiglottis; 8. C2; 9. Anterior arch of C1.)

102. (c) Structure 2 in Figure 6 is the posterior arch of the atlas (C1). **BU**

103. (b) Structure 3 in Figure 6 is the spinous process. **BA**

104. (a) Structure 4 in Figure 6 is the esosphagus. **BU**

105. (a) Structure 7 in Figure 6 is the epiglottis. **BU**

106. (b) The conus medullaris is the lower portion of the spinal cord. **BU**

107. (b) The conus ends at the T12/L1 level. **BU**

108. (b) The individual nerve roots leave the conus and progress downward through the lower lumbar canal. This is called the cauda equina. **BU**

109. (a) A condition in which the cord is pulled lower than its natural level is called a tethered cord. **ST**

110. (a) CSF is dark on T1- and bright on T2-weighted images. **BU**

111. (c) A patient with a pituitary disorder may display irregular menses or experience leaking from her breasts, a conditon known as galactorrhea. **TA**

112. (b) Because the vertebral bodies contain marrow, they usually display a bright appearance. Fractures or re-

placement of the marrow by infection or neoplasm cause less signal intensity. **BU**

113. (a) The axial plane best demonstrates both the dorsal and ventral nerve roots. **BU**

114. (b) Structure 4 in Figure 7 is CSF. **BU**

(Key to Figure 7: 1. Cerebellar tonsil; 2. Posterior arch C1; 3. Spinal cord; 4. CSF; 5. Spinous ligament; 6. Venous plexus; 7. Anterior longitudinal ligament (ALL); 8. Posterior longitudinal ligament (PLL).)

115. (b) Structure 7 in Figure 7 is the anterior longitudinal ligament (ALL). **MO**

116. (c) Structure 1 in Figure 8 is the first thorocic vertebrae.

(Key to Figure 8: 1. 1st thoracic vertebrae; 2. C2.)

117. (b) Structue 1 in Figure 9 is the nerve root. **MO**

(Key to Figure 9: 1. Nerve root; 2. Transverse process; 3. Lamina; 4. Spinous process.)

118. (b) Structure 2 in Figure 9 is the transverse process. **MO**

119. (b) Structure 3 in Figure 9 is the lamina. **BU**

120. (d) Structure 4 in Figure 9 is the spinous process. **MO**

121. (d) Healthy disc does not enhance after the administration of gadolinium. **BR**

122. (c) A healthy nucleus pulposus generally displays a bright signal intensity on T2-weighted images. **BU**

123. (b) The soft inner portion of the disc is known as the nucleus pulposus. **AP**

124. (b) Structure 2 in Figure 10 is the cauda equina. **BU**

(Key to Figure 10: 1. Spinous process; 2. Cauda equina; 3. Venous plexus; 4. Annulus fibrosus; 5. PLL; 6. ALL; 7. Nucleus pulposus; 8. Sacrum.)

125. (c) Structure 5 in Figure 10 is the posterior longitudinal ligament (PLL). **MO**

126. (c) The tough exterior of the vertebral disc is known as the annulus fibrosus. **AP** (Number 4 in Figure 10)

127. (a) Structure 3 in Figure 10 displays the venous plexus or basivertebral vein. **MO**

128. (b) The brachial plexus is at the C4-T2 level. **NE**

129. (a) Nerve roots located in the T2-L4 area are considered the lumbar plexus. **NE**

130. (a) Lung tissue is typically black on both T1- and T2–weighted sequences. **BU**

131. (a) The right ventricle is the most anterior chamber of the heart as seen on cross sectional images. **BU**

132. (a) The left atrium is the most posteriorly located of the heart. **BU**

133. (c) The left ventricle is known by its thick muscular walls. **BU**

134. (a) The heart should be imaged during its quiet phase–diastole. **POTT**

135. (c) The carina is the level at which the left and right pulmonary bronchi bifurcate. **TA**

136. (a) The pulmonary artery is the only artery that carries deoxygenated blood. **AP**

137. (c) The body coil is used to visualize the thorax. **ST**

138. (d) Respiratory gating is helpful in suppressing motion caused by breathing. Use of either the cardiac or peripheral gating helps to limit motion from the beating of the heart in the thorax area. **POTT**

139. (b) It is important to trigger off of the R wave. **POTT**

140. (b) Structure 2 in Figure 11 is the muscular left ventricle. **BU**

(Key to Figure 11: 1.Left atrium; 2. Left ventricle; 3. Right ventricle; 4. Right atrium.)

141. (d) Structure 4 in Figure 11 is the right atrium. **BU**

142. (b) Structure 3 in Figure 11 is the right ventricle. **BU**

143. (b) The liver is the largest organ in the abdominal cavity. **AP**

144. (b) Fat, the pancreas, and spleen are all gray on T2–weighted images. **BU**

145. (a) THe transverse (axial) plane best displays the pancreas. **BU**

146. (b) The azygos veins drain the thoracic wall and the posterior abdominal wall. **AP**

147. (a) A chemical shift artifact is the result of fat and water protons resonating at different frequencies. **POTT**

148. (d) Some of the organs located behind the peritoneal sac (retroperitoneally) are the kidneys, pancreas, duodenum, and lymph nodes. **AP**
149. (a) Structure 1 in Figure 12 is the right ventricle. **BU**

    (Key to Figure 12: 1. Right ventricle; 2. Aorta; 3. Left atrium.)
150. (d) All three issues are important when imaging the breast. **WO**
151. (c) In order to more clearly define a mass in the breast, the administration of contrast is necessary. T1–weighted images with fat saturation post contrast define a mass while suppressing the fatty tissue of the breast. **WO**
152. (a) Structure 3 in Figure 13 is the psoas muscle. **MO**

    (Key to Figure 13: 1. Bladder; 2. Ilium; 3. Psoas muscle; 4. Femoral head; 5. Greater trochanter; 6. Gluteal muscles; 7. Obturator internus; 8. Obturator externus.)
153. (c) Structure 5 in Figure 13 is the greater trochanter. **MO**
154. (d) Structure 7 in Figure 13 is the obturator internus muscle. **MO**
155. (a) Structure 2 in Figure 13 is the ilium. **MO**
156. (d) Structure 1 in Figure 14 is the bladder. **MO**

    (Key to Figure 14: 1. Bladder; 2. Pubic symphysis; 3. Prostate; 4. Endorectal coil; 5. 5th lumbar vertebrae; 6. Aorta; 7. Coccyx; 8. Sacrum.)
157. (d) Structure 2 in Figure 14 is the pubic symphysis. **MO**
158. (a) Structure 3 in Figure 14 is the prostate. **MO**
159. (a) Structure 4 in Figure 14 is the endorectal coil. **MO**
160. (b) Structure 6 in Figure 14 is the thoracic aorta. **MO**
161. (b) The body coil is typically used to display the pelvis on an adult. **ST**
162. (d) The endorectal coil is used to scan the prostate. **ST**
163. (d) An IR sequence is useful in showing a bone bruise, especially in the knee area. **ST**
164. (d) There are no known contraindications for gadolinium. **OM,MA,PR**
165. (a) Structure 1 in Figure 15 is the liver. **MO**

(Key to Figure 15: 1. Liver; 2. Gallbladder; 3. Portal vein; 4. Stomach; 5. Aorta; 6. Spleen; 7. Inferior vena cava.)

166. (b) Structure 2 in Figure 15 is the gallbladder. **MO**
167. (d) Structure 3 in Figure 15 is the portal vein. **MO**
168. (c) Structure 4 in Figure 15 is the stomach. **MO**
169. (a) Structure 6 in Figure 15 is the spleen. **MO**
170. (b) Structure 7 in Figure 15 is the inferior vena cava. **MO**
171. (a) Structure 5 in Figure 16 is the renal cortex. **MO**

(Key to Figure 16: 1. Inferior vena cava; 2. Superior mesenteric vein; 3. Superior mesenteric artery; 4. Aorta; 5. Renal cortex.)

172. (a) Structure 4 in Figure 16 is the aorta. **MO**
173. (c) Structure 3 in Figure 16 is the superior mesenteric artery. **MO**
174. (d) All of the answers are synonymous with 0.2 ml/kg, which is the effective dose for gadolinium. **POTT**
175. (b) Eighty percent of the gadolinium is excreted by the kidneys in three hours. **POTT**
176. (d) A surface coil, which produces better SNR, is used to display the shoulder. **BU**
177. (d) The 3-inch surface coil is used to view the temporo-mandibular joint. **ST**
178. (b) A kinematic device is used to display the range of motion on the TMJ. **ST**
179. (c) Structure 3 in Figure 17 is the external meatus. **MO**

(Key to Figure 17: 1. Temporal lobe; 2. Condyle of the mandible; 3. External auditory canal; 4. Meniscus.)

180. (a) Structure 4 in Figure 17 is the TMJ disk or the TMJ meniscus. **BA**
181. (d) The landmark when scanning the brain is at the nasion. Siemens Users Manual
182. (a) Structure 1 in Figure 18 is the deltoid muscle. **MO**

(Key to Figure 18: 1. Deltoid muscle; 2. Humeral head; 3. Glenoid; 4. Labrum; 5. Supraspinatus muscle; 6. Acromion; 7. Supraspinatus tendon.)

183. (d) Structure 2 in Figure 18 is the humeral head. **MO**
184. (c) Structure 3 in Figure 18 is the glenoid fossa. **MO**

185. (a) Structure 4 in Figure 18 is the labrum. **MO**
186. (b) Structure 5 in Figure 18 is the supraspinatus muscle. **MO**
187. (a) Structure 6 in Figure 18 is the acromion. **MO**
188. (b) Figure 18 is an off-axis coronal projection. **MO**
189. (c) Structure 19 is an off-axis sagittal projection. **MO**

(Key to Figure 19:1. Clavicle; 2. Acromion; 3. Coracoid process; 4. Humeral head; 5. Supraspinatus muscle; 6. Supraspinatus tendon.)

190. (b) Structure 1 in Figure 19 is the acromion. **MO**
191. (c) The supraspinatus, infraspinatus, teres minor, and subscapularis make up the rotator cuff. **ST**
192. (b) An extremity coil provides excellent SNR of the knee. **BU**
193. (c) A natural, 15° external rotation of the foot will best demonstrate the anterior cruciate ligament of the knee.
194. (c) Figure 20 displays a coronal projection of the knee. **MO**

(Key to Figure 20: 1. Lateral meniscus; 2. Femoral condyle; 3. Posterior cruciate ligament; 4. Tibia; 5. Tibial spine; 6. Collateral ligament.)

195. (c) Structure 3 in Figure 20 is the posterior cruciate ligament. **MO**
196. (c) Structure 4 in Figure 20 is the tibia. **MO**
197. (a) Structure 1 in Figure 20 is the lateral meniscus. **MO**
198. (b) Structure 6 in Figure 21 is the quadriceps tendon. **MO**
199. (a) Structure 1 in Figure 21 is the patella. **MO**

(Key to Figure 21: 1. Patella; 2. Femur; 3. Posterior horn of the lateral meniscus; 4. Tibia; 5. Patellar tendon; 6. Quadriceps tendon; 7. Fibula; 8. Gastrocnemius muscle.)

200. (c) Structure 4 in Figure 21 is the tibia. **MO**
201. (b) Structure 7 in Figure 21 is the fibula. **MO**
202. (a) Structure 5 in Figure 21 is the patellar tendon. **MO**
203. (b) Structure 1 in Figure 22 is the radius. **BU**

(Key to Figure 22: 1. Radius; 2. Scaphoid; 3. Triquetral; 4. Triangular fibrocartilage; 5. Capitate.)

204. (c) Structure 4 in Figure 22 is the triangular fibrocartilage. **BU**

205. (a) Imaging in the axial plane best demonstrates compression of the carpal tunnel area. **BU**

206. (a) AVN is a condition in which a portion of the bone becomes necrotic because of the lack of a neccessary blood supply. **ST**

207. (d) Structure 1 in Figure 23 is the olecranon. **STO**

    (Key to Figure 23: 1. Olecranon; 2. Coronoid; 3. Radial head; 4. Capitellum.)

208. (a) Structure 3 in Figure 23 is the radial head. **STO**

209. (d) Structure 2 in Figure 23 is the coronoid. **STO**

210. (c) Structure 4 in Figure 23 is the capitellum. **STO**

211. (d) TR is the time from the application of the initial RF pulse to the next RF pulse applied to the same slice. **WE**

212. (b) TE is the time from the application of the initial RF pulse to the peak of the return signal induced in the coil. **WE**

213. (c) A long TE is used to give fat and water time to decay. Long TR sequences allow time for the T1 of fat and water to fully recover, therefore image contrast will be based on T2 decay changes. **WE**

214. (a) The 180° RF pulse compensates for T2 and T2* dephasing that occur immediately following the application of the 90° RF pulse. **WE**

215. (b) The preparation pulse serves to flip the spins from the positive longitudinal plane 180° into the negative longitudinal direction creating a larger dynamic range in the T1 relaxation process. **WO**

216. (d) A partial flip angle of less than 90° is used to shorten the T1 relaxation time, shortening TR and the scan time. A gradient reversal application is needed to refocus spins in the transverse plane. **WO**

217. (b) Only protons in fat and water (mobile protons) are measured in MR. **LU**

218. (a) FSE sequences use a 90° RF pulse followed by a train of 180° RF pulses and produce true T2–weighted images. **WE**

219. (b) Presaturation pulses produce a signal void by pre-saturating the flowing spins before they move into the imaging volume. **WE**

220. (c) The time it takes to rephase net magnetization after the application of the 180° RF pulse equals the time the net magnetization vector takes to dephase after the 90° RF pulse. **WE**

221. (c) The time it takes to rephase net magnetization after the application of the 180° RF pulse equals the time the net magnetization vector takes to dephase after the 90° RF pulse. **WE**

222. (a) Lengthening TE increases the amount of T2 relaxation that has occurred over time. The overall contrast mechanism for T2 contrast is TE. **WO**

223. (c) In GRE pulse sequences TR and flip angle control the amount of T1 relaxation that occurs before the next RF pulse is applied. This is saturation. **WE**

224. (b) Flow signal enhancement is increased in GRE sequences. Low TRs are used to saturate stationary nuclei such that flowing nuclei appear to have a higher signal. These sequences are said to be flow sensitive. **WE**

225. (c) The decaying sinusoidal waveform after the 90° RF pulse is known as free induction decay, (FID) and is due primarily from T2* relaxation effects. **WO**

226. (b) The gradient reversal application is not as effective as the 180° RF pulse in refocusing spins and is therefore sensitive to magnetic field inhomogeneity or T2* effects. **LU**

227. (d) The shorter the TE time, the more spins are still in phase to return a strong signal. **WO**

228. (d) Gradient spoilers are placed subsequent to the collection of the echo to dephase any remaining transverse magnetization. This allows only longitudinal magnetization to contribute to the next RF pulse. **WO**

229. (d) Long TR sequences allow sufficient time for most tissues to return to the longitudinal plane. The short TE allows for signal return before significant T2 de-

cay has occurred. These factors increase the proton density weighting of the image. **WO**

230. (d) In 3DFT sequences, a slice encoding process is added to the pulse sequence design and is applied similar to phase encoding. This added design increases scan time by the number of slices requested. The formula for 3DFT scan time is:
TR (sec) x Npe x NEX x Nslices / 60 sec. **WO**

231. (d) Partial saturation pulse sequences begin with a 90° RF pulse and is then followed by the collection of the echo. **WE**

232. (b) Reducing the Npe reduces scan time and resolution but does not directly affect image contrast. **WE**

233. (c) T2 dephasing causes the peak signal for spin echoes to be less than the initial FID signal. **WE**

234. (c) Gradients are used to rephase transverse magnetization so that both longitudinal and transverse signals contribute to the image. **WO**

235. (c) An SE pulse sequence is defined as a sequence of events where a 90° RF pulse is followed by a 180° RF pulse and then the signal is measured. **WO**

236. (b) Hahn echoes are formed from two successive RF pulses, other than 90° and 180°. **EL**

237. (c) TR determines the interval at which the pulse sequences repeat and therefore directly affects acquisition time. **WE**

238. (d) Steady state is a condition in which the TR is shorter than the T1 and T2 times of the tissues. Therefore there is no time for the transverse magnetization to decay before the pulse sequence is repeated. The flip angle and the TR maintain steady state, which holds the longitudinal and transverse components of magnetization and the net magnetization vector steady during the acquisition. **WE**

239. (a) Velocity of blood flow is defined by the distance traveled between the positive and negative lobe of the velocity-encoding gradient. **EL**

240. (b) High-flow and turbulence cause a decrease or void in signal intensity. Diastolic pseudogating causes an increase in signal intensity. **LU**

241. (b) The shorter the flip angle the lower the amount of RF transmitted and therefore the lower the amount of signal received that lowers SNR. **WO**

242. (d) Incoherent pulse sequences use a GRE to rephase only the FID portion of the SE. The SE portion is spoiled and is not sampled. **WE**

243. (d) IR pulse sequences flip net magnetization vector 180° or twice the dynamic range possible with spin echoes. **WO**

244. (a) T2 contrast is affected by changes in TE time. Spin density increases with increases in TR. SNR decreases because the lowering of TR reduces the amount of longitudinal magnetization allowed to return signal. **WO**

245. (c) It takes four times the amount of power of a 90° RF pulse to produce a 180° RF pulse; $(ø/\,90°)^2 = RF$ power deposited. **MI**

246. (c) TI is the time of inversion; the length of time longitudinal magnetization is allowed to relax from the negative z-plane before applying the 90° RF pulse. **LU**

247. (c) SNR is proportional to $\sqrt{NEX}$ and $\dfrac{1}{\sqrt{(received\ bandwidth)}}$. **WE**

248. (a) Gradient reversals change the polarity of the spins causing those spins that have sped up as a result of the positive gradient to slow down and those that have slowed due to the negative gradient to speed up. This is unlike the 180° RF pulse that flips the spin's direction. **WO**

249. (a) A 45° flip angle has 1/4 the power of a 90° (or unit). Since a CSE sequence employs a 90° and a 180° pulse, the total power is 5 units of 90° power; a 180° RF pulse is 4 times the power of a 90°. In a GRE only one 45° RF pulse is used, which is 1/4 of a unit (90° RF power). Therefore a 45° RF GRE is 1/20th or 5% the power used in a CSE. **MI**

250. (b) The data collected in the phase and frequency direction of k- space is split into positive and negative portions. These portions are mirrors of one another.

If only part of one portion is collected in the frequency direction, the other can be conjugated or filled in. This is called fractional echo. **WE**

251. (d) Reducing the bandwidth results in less noise being sampled relative to signal, increasing SNR. Reducing the bandwidth increases the sampling time which also increases the minimum TE. **WE**

252. (b) Presaturation pulses are used to presaturate flowing spins prior to entry into the region of interest, which in turn reduces flow artifacts. **WO**

253. (a) For effectiveness presaturation pulses must be placed prior to the excitation pulse to presaturate flowing spins prior to RF excitation. **WE**

254. (b) The central lines of k-space are filled with shallow phase encoding gradients that result in higher signal amplitude and low spatial resolution collected. **WE**

255. (a) The range of frequencies comprising the receive bandwidth is sampled by the readout or frequency encoding gradient. **WE**

256. (c) 1 T = 10,000 G; 1T = 1000 mT; 10,000G = 1000 mT; 10mm = 1 cm; 10 mT/m = 1.0 G/cm. **LU**

257. (c) Rise time is the time required for the gradient to go from no power to full or maximum power. The faster the rise time, the more efficient the gradient coil and power supply are and the more capable they are of acquiring data in rapid time sequences. **LU**

258. (d) Because of random noise collected during the echo, the SNR is increased by the square root of 2. Therefore doubling the NEX increases the SNR 1.41 times. **WE**

259. (a) The outer lines of k-space are filled using high amplitude gradients that produce high resolution image quality with low signal return. **WE**

260. (d) NEX controls the amount of data that is stored in each line of k-space. Each line of k-space uses a specific gradient amplitude each time data is placed there. **WE**

261. (a) Reducing the bandwidth increases SNR but also increases sampling time based on the Nyquist theo-

rem. The longer the sampling time, the longer the frequency encoding gradient must remain on. **WE**

262. (b) When sinc-shaped RF pulse profiles are transformed, the resulting slice profile is square in shape, permitting nearly contiguous slices. **LU**

263. (c) SNR is proportional to $\frac{1}{\sqrt{Npe}}$ (phase encodes), and is proportional to the slice thickness and the flip angle. **WE**

264. (a) In a 3D sequence's initial RF, a shallow slice select gradient is applied. This will not allow slice selection to occur. Therefore to encode slices the slice select gradient must be turned on in the same manner as the phase encode gradient, that is, the slice select gradient must be turned on for as many slices as are requested. **WO**

265. (b) Since only tissues having recovered a substantial portion of their magnetization can fully respond to subsequent pulses, this causes saturation of certain tissues (those that cannot recover fast enough) and a loss of signal intensity. **WO**

266. (a) 3D sequences have limited FOV and scan times that are not short enough for breath-hold sequences. Short TEs are necessary to minimize flow-turbulence-related artifacts. With very short T1 tissues, saturation of the spins is often difficult to maintain, reducing the effectiveness of the sequence for background suppression. **WO**

267. (d) All of the statements are true regarding vascular imaging and need no further explanation. **WO**

268. (b) MIP produces a projection image with signals from overlapping structures superimposed on one 2D projection image. A ray passing through vascular anatomy should retain a high maximum intensity as it encounters a bright blood vessel; and a ray passing through background tissue should only record a low saturated maximum intensity. **WO**

269. (b) MRA is a record of blood flow, not a record of the vessel or the tissues itself, so any disturbances in flow is recorded as a change in signal. **WO**

270. (a) Normal human peak systolic flow velocites vary with age, cardiac output and anatomical site. The normal lower and upper values are 20-175 cm/sec, however for certain pathologic conditions, velocities can increase up to 400 cm/sec. **EL**

271. (c) The ascending aorta has the highest peak systolic blood flow because of its proximity to the heart and size of the vessel. **EL**

272. (b) Laminar flow. In theory, the distribution of velocities in a perfectly straight, nonbranching vessel with nonpulsatile flow, should be parabolic with peak velocities at the center of the lumen. However, because of the elasticity and pulsatility effects in the real world, the flow profile can be more blunted. **EL**

273. (d) Also called flow eddies, vortex flow frequently occurs at vascular bifurcation and distal to areas of stenosis. Vortex flow is composed of slowly moving currents and streamlines that are not random but are often countercurrent to the main flow direction. **EL**

274. (b) TOF effects. Unsaturated blood flows into an imaging volume that has been partially saturated by multiple RF. The new signal (from unsaturated blood) is higher. As the flow penetrates into the imaging volume, only the higher velocities at the center of the lumen demonstrate enhancement. High-velocity signal loss is a TOF effect in which spins flow out of the slice before completing the 90° and 180° RF stimulation. **EL**

275. (c) TEs of 30/60/90/120 msec are evenly spaced. Loss of signal occurs after the odd echoes (30 and 90 msec) due to dephasing. Increased signal caused by spin rephasing occurs from the even numbered echoes (60 and 120 msec). **EL**

276. (d) Turbulence takes place when blood velocities exceed a critical threshold or when vascular morphology creates a disruption of the laminar flow state. Turbulence, is seen in the aorta, at the vascular bifurcations, and distal to areas of stenosis. **EL**

277. (b) Saturation results in a progressive signal decrease in the tissue signal until a steady state is reached between the longitudinal recovery of the tissue and the action of the RF pulses. **EL**

278. (a) Turbulent flow takes place when blood velocities exceed a critical threshold or when vascular morphology creates the disruption the laminar flow state. Turbulent flow is seen in the aorta, at the vascular bifurcation, and distal to areas of stenosis. **EL**

279. (c) Since the gradient magnetic field is proportional to position, the induced phase shift is then also proportional to position. **POTC**

280. (b) Laminar means that the velocity of blood at the vessel wall is zero and the velocity profile across the vessel is parabolic, peaking in the center of the vessel. **POTC**

281. (b) TOF effects in MRI arise from the movement of longitudinal magnetization during a relatively long period. **POTC**

282. (c) The phase of transverse magnetization is extremely sensitive to movement along a magnetic field gradient. Blood motion over a distance of less than a pixel during a gradient pulse is sufficient to cause measurable phase shifts. **POTC**

283. (b) TE affects T2 weighting, as T2 relaxation is TE dependent. As TE is increased, T2 weighting increases. **WO**

284. (d) T1 is TR dependent. As TR decreases, the amount of T1 contrast displayed increases, differentiating between tissues with short and long T1 relaxation times. **WO**

285. (d) To form an SE requires the application of a 90° RF pulse and a 180° RF pulse. Each subsequent 180° RF pulse after the initial 90° RF pulse produces another echo, totaling six, until the 90° pulse is applied again. **WO**

286. (a) The echo with the highest signal will be the echo collected at the shortest TE time. As TE lengthens, more spin-spin interactions occur which causes dephasing and thus signal loss. **WO**

287. (d) The 180° RF pulse refocuses spins in the transverse plane and allows for rephasing and maximum signal return. **WO**

288. (d) If steep gradient slopes are used to produce thin slices, fine matrices or small FOV are also usually selected. **WE**

289. (d) Increasing the FOV requires an increase in either the matrix size or the pixel size. Increasing the slab thickness requires an increase in the area excited by the RF pulse. All cause an increase in signal. Increasing TE decreases signal due to T2 spin dephasing. **WO**

290. (a) Chemical shift misregistration presents with a void of signal on the high-frequency side and an addition of signal on the low-frequency side of organs due to the 3.5 ppm difference in precessional frequencies between fat and water. **WO**

291. (b) T2 tissue characteristics are enhanced or limited by the length of time allowed for the spins to dephase before collection of the echo. The parameter, TE, determines the length of time allowed before listening to the echo. **WO**

292. (c) The amount of T1 relaxation is dependent on the length of TR. The shorter the TR, the less time long T1 tissues have to return their signal, leaving tissues that have short relaxation times to return signal. The TR is significant in determining the desired about of T1 relaxation prior to another RF excitation. **WO**

293. (d) T2 decay occurs with subsequent echoes. T2 decay is increased with spin-spin interactions, magnetic susceptibility, and magnetic field inhomogeneities. **WO**

294. (c) Symmetric echoes. Constant velocity flow through a constant gradient increases phase shift quadratically. Phase dispersions are lower on even-numbered echoes than on odd-numbered echoes. Even echo rephasing is typically seen on symmetric echoes due to vessel flow within an imaging plane. **EL**

295. (c) Presaturation pulses help to eliminate both patient breathing motion and flow artifacts from blood flow. **WE**

296. (a) Reducing the number of averages reduces the number of times that data is collected. The less data collected, the lower the SNR. **WE**

297. (d) Measurements collect signal and noise. Noise is random and will affect the proportionality of the SNR. **EL**

298. (d) VENC is critical to the performance of the MRA pulse sequence. If set too high, the range of flow imaged does not encompass the proper number of phase shifts to record the data accurately; signal-to-noise decreases and slow flow in vessels is difficult to see. **EL**

299. (d) The FOV is comprised of voxels. Reducing the FOV by a factor of two reduces the voxel on both directions by a factor of two, reducing the volume by a total factor of four. **WE**

300. (c) As the receive bandwidth decreases, the sampling time increases. An increase in sample time increases SNR. **WE**

301. (c) Receive bandwidth is inversely proportional to sample time. The lower the receive bandwidth, the higher the SNR. **WE**

302. (b) Pixel = FOV / matrix; FOV = matrix x pixel. **WE**

303. (b) TR affects T1 contrast and proton concentration. Although T2-weighted images use a long TR, it is TE that affects T2 contrast. **WO**

304. (a) Loosely bound hydrogen takes a longer time to dephase and remains brighter for a longer period of time. **WO**

305. (c) TR and flip angle control the amount of T1 relaxation allowed to regrow before being excited again by an RF pulse. **WE**

306. (b) T2 is TE dependent. The amount of T2 relaxation that occurs before the next excitation is dependent on the amount of time allowed from the RF excitation pulse to the sample of the echo. **WO**

307. (a) Magnetic field relates to magnetic force. As the field strength decreases, so does the magnetic force that holds the spins in the longitudinal plane. The less force holding the spins in the longitudinal plane, the less power (RF) necessary to tip it out. The less power transmitted, the shorter the amount of time to relax back. **WO**

308. (c) The local inhomogeneities within solids cause rapid dephasing of the transverse magnetization (spin-spin interactions). **WO**

309. (b) Protein binding effects affect the rate of molecular motion and the efficiency of the molecule to relax back to the lattice. This has an effect on the relaxation time and causes an effect on image appearance. **LU**

310. (d) Signal-to-noise is a ratio of the amount of signal collected to the amount of random noise collected. **WE**

311. (d) Noise depends on the build of the patient, the area under examination, the inherent noise of the system, occurs at all frequencies and is also random in time. **WE**

312. (d) Virtually all imaging parameters affect the amount of signal and noise collected in each image. **WE**

313. (d) Volume elements (or voxels) are determined by the pixel size and the slice thickness and contain signal from a volume of tissue. **WE**

314. (d) Doubling the FOV means doubling the length and width of the matrix or the pixel. If the area is doubled in each direction, the overall effect is a quadrupling of the area and therefore a quadrupling of the SNR. **WE**

315. (b) The phase encoding gradient for each slice is turned on for as many matrix steps as desired (256) times the number of NEX (2) chosen for a total of 512. **WO**

316. (c) Magnetic susceptibility is determined by the electron configuration of the atom. The orbital angular momentum of the electron is much greater than the dipole generated by the nucleus. Although MR resonance depends on the nucleus, the overall mag-

netic environment that also affects the image is based on the presence of paired or unpaired electrons. **LU**

317. (d) The transmit bandwidth determines the range of frequencies used to transmit RF into the patient and determines the thickness of the slice based on gradient slope. **LU**

318. (b) Receive bandwidth is inversely proportional to sampling time. **LU**

319. (c) TR has a direct effect on acquisition time. All other parameters can be manipulated independent of TR. **WO**

320. (d) SNR is affected by all imaging parameters. With increases in pixel size and acquisition SNR increases. By reducing the bandwidth, SNR also increases. **WO**

321. (b) The TR is determined by the R-R interval which is dictated by the patient's heart rate. **WO**

322. (b) For heavily T1-weighted images using IR pulses requires that the TI be approximately 1/4 TR to allow for contrast differentiation between tissues that have short and long T1 relaxation times. **WO**

323. (a) T2 is TE dependent The longer the TE, the more dependence on T2 tissue characteristics to create image contrast. **WO**

324. (a) To presaturate spins that may flow into the region of interest the presaturation pulse must be applied prior to the initial RF pulse. **WO**

325. (c) If the TE is reduced, the dependence on T2 for image contrast decreases. With short TE times less T2 dephasing occurs increasing proton concentration. **WO**

326. (c) TR and TE primarily affect SNR. TI determines the amount of T1 relaxation during the pulse sequence and therefore the contrast of the image. **WO**

327. (a) Sixty-three percent of the regrowth of the longitudinal magnetization is defined as T1 relaxation time. **WE**

328. (c) TR and flip angle control the amount of saturation of the tissues. Reducing TR and flip angle reduces the amount of saturation. **WE**

329. (a) Receive bandwidth refers to the range of received frequencies from the FOV. These frequencies are manipulated by the frequency encoding or read out gradient. **WE**

330. (c) The smaller the receive bandwidth, the narrower the FOV. To maintain the image size, the gradient amplitude must be lowered, increasing SNR. **LU**

331. (c) Slice thickness is manipulated by adjusting the gradient amplitude or the transmit bandwidth. **LU**

332. (a) The lower the receive bandwidth, the longer the frequency gradient must be on to sample the FOV. Receive bandwidth is inversely proportional to sampling time. **LU**

333. (c) FOV reduction causes reduction in both the length and width of the FOV. This reduction has a four-fold decrease affect on the size of the voxel volume. **WE**

334. (c) The time between 90° RF pulses (TR) is also referred to as the duty cycle because it represents the total amount of time required for each view or phase encoding step in image formation. **LU**

335. (c) If the chosen TR is less than the T2 relaxation of the tissue, transverse magnetization is not allowed to fully dephase which will, with subsequent RF pulses, create a steady state. **WE**

336. (b) Sixty-nine percent of the T1 of the tissue is the point where the tissue intersects the transverse plane. This is called the null point of the tissue, and it is at this point that there is no net magnetization. **WO**

337. (c) The number of echoes, sixteen, determine the number of lines of k-space filled with each TR. **WE**

338. (c) An increase in the slab or the number of slices increases SNR in 3D sequences. **WE**

339. (c) The first moment of flow is velocity. **POTC**

340. (b) The second moment of flow is acceleration. **POTC**

341. (b) The effective TE is placed on the central lines of k-space where contrast and signal-to-noise will have the most affect on image quality. **WE**

342. (c) GRE contrast is based on T1 tissue characteristics. There is no true T2 information gathered during GRE sequences because there is no RF pulse (180°) to refocus the spins. **WO**

343. (d) Gradient pulses subsequent to the echo spoil the rest of the transverse magnetization, which makes the gradient phase dispersions nonzero and provide more T1 dependence during the next RF and echo. **WO**

344. (d) Rephased GRE rephase the transverse magnetization, which will preserve it, contributing both T1 and T2 tissues to the next pulse and resulting in an increase in T2* dependence. **WO**

345. (a) The formula for the length of scan is TR x Npe x NEX. **WO**

346. (c) In FSE sequences, the number of echoes per TR used to create the image is the echo train length (ETL). **WO**

347. (c) The larger the ETL the longer it takes before the last echo is collected and the less dead time is available to collect additional slices. **WO**

348. (d) Reducing the echo train spacing (ETS) will result in a increase in the allowed number of slices, improves contrast control, and will reduce blurring. **WO**

349. (d) 3D SE pulse sequences use a phase encoding function in the slice select direction (gradient) to slice encode slices from a 3D slab. **WO**

350. (c) The basic equation for signal strength in a SE sequence leads to a maximum SNR per unit of scan time at a TR of 1.26 times the T1 for the single tissue being considered. **WO**

351. (b) Net transverse magnetization is obtained when the net magnetic vector is flipped 90° into the transverse plane. **WE**

352. (d) The 180° RF pulse is a refocusing pulse and flips the transverse magnetization 180° into the opposite direction of the transverse plane. **WE**

353. (a) Short TR acquisitions differentiate tissue with long and short T1 relaxation times, increasing T1 contrast. A short TE minimizes the amount of T2 relaxation that is allowed to contribute to overall image contrast. **WE**

354. (b) As FOV is reduced, either pixel size or matrix size is reduced, possibly both. Reducing the pixel or matrix size increases spatial resolution, minimizing partial voluming effects. **WO**

355. (b) This is a STIR sequence, indicated by the short TI time. This type of sequence provides fat suppression. **WO**

356. (c) By definition an SE pulse sequence is a series of RF pulse events in which an initial 90° RF pulse is followed by at least one 180° RF pulse. **WO**

357. (b) In 3D FT pulse sequences the slices are first acquired as a slab using a broad amplitude slice select gradient. Slices are then encoded to whatever slice thickness is desired by slice encoding or repeating applications of the slice select gradient. **WO**

358. (d) A gap is often required to reduce the amount of cross-talk between adjacent slices providing more coverage. Since cross-talk is reduced signal-to-noise will increase. **WE**

359. (c) Long T2 tissues maintain transverse magnetization for longer times and therefore maintain strong signal return. **WE**

360. (b) The narrower the bandwidth, the less the area excited by the RF pulse. Combined with steep gradient this produces thin slices. **WE**

361. (c) The steepness of the frequency encoding gradient determines the range of frequencies recorded as an MR signal that create the FOV. **WE**

362. (d) The sample time is the length of time the frequency encoding gradient is active to sample the echo. **WE**

363. (c) The Nyquist theorem states that any signal must be sampled at least twice per cycle to represent it accurately. The sampling time, sampling rate, and receive bandwidth are all linked by the Nyquist theorem. In addition, enough cycles must occur dur-

ing the sampling time to achieve enough frequency samples. **WE**

364. (b) The sample time is inversely proportional to sampling rate and to the receive bandwidth. **WE**

365. (a) Broad transmit bandwidths are necessary to excite a larger area or thicker slices. **WE**

366. (c) By definition TR is the length of time between successive RF pulses applied to the same slice (time to repeat). **WE**

367. (b) Matrix steps is determined by the number of phase and frequency steps chosen. The matrix size is then determined based on the size of each step in each direction. **WE**

368. (c) The proton density or concentration is most responsible for the overall signal of an image. The more protons returning a signal the higher the signal return. **WE**

369. (b) Intravoxel dephasing occurs when spins within the same voxel have different spin phase. The dephasing causes a loss of signal. **WE**

370. (b) $\dfrac{\sqrt{original\,BW}}{\sqrt{new\,BW}} = \dfrac{\sqrt{8}}{\sqrt{4}} = \dfrac{\sqrt{2}}{\sqrt{1}} = \sqrt{2} = 1.41$, which is a 40% increase or improvement in SNR. **WE**

371. (d) new FOV x/original FOVx = 160/360 = .5
new FOV y/original FOVy = 160/360 = .5
.5 x .5 = 0.25.
The amount of SNR for a 16 cm FOV would be .25 of the 36 cm FOV.
SNR = $\sqrt{NEX}$, then NEX = SNR^2;
$(1/0.25)^2 = 4^2 = 16$ times scan time. **WE**

372. (d) The smaller matrix (Npe) divided by the larger matrix (Npe) 192/256 = .75; $\sqrt{.75}$ = .87 or 87%. **WE**

373. (c) Sample rate is directly proportional to receive bandwidth and indirectly proportional to sample time. **WE**

374. (b) Any parameter that changes the size of the voxel increases or decreases SNR. **WE**

375. (b) Square root of the change; 128/256 = .5; $\sqrt{.5}$ = .707 or 71%. **WE**

376. (b) An increase in TE increases the amount of T2 dephasing that decreases SNR. **WE**

377. (c) TE is the length of time from the initial RF pulse to the middle of the listening window for the echo. **WE**

378. (b) The RF pulse waveform determines the efficiency of the RF pulse to excite the slices. The more square the RF pulse profile is, the less cross-talk results. **WE**

379. (a) Reducing the sample rate means that data is collected at a reduced interval, requiring a longer time to collect the data and increasing the sample time. **WE**

380. (b) Long TR, Long TE (SE) creates T2-weighted images. **WO**

381. (b) 2D volumetric imaging using this acquisition method and is the most common type used. **WE**

382. (b) TR x Npe x NEX / 60,000 msec = 12.8 min. **WE**

383. (d) Only a 90° RF pulse followed by a 180° RF pulse will produce true T2-weighted image. **WE**

384. (c) An increase in TR increases scan time which will potentially increase motion artifacts. **WO**

385. (c) The TI or interpulse time is the main contrast controlling mechanism. TI determines when the data acquisition window starts to acquire data. This affects where on the relaxation curve the data is acquired. **WO**

386. (b) Fast GRE sequences acquire all the data per image each time the data acquisition window is turned on, per TR. **WO**

387. (b) 240 mm / 256 = .937 or .94 mm. **WE**

388. (c) 90° RF followed by two 180° RF pulses - CSE - double echo. **WO**

389. (a) Images acquired at a short time during longitudinal relaxation maximize T1 image contrast creating T1–weighted images. **WO**

390. (c) 3D sequences do not slice select with RF, rather slice encode for as many slices as are requested using the slice select gradient in a fashion similar to phase encoding. **WO**

391. (d) The dimensions of k-space are similar to a matrix and have a phase and frequency axis comprising a number of lines or steps. **WO**

392. (d) Spoiled GRE. The extra gradient pulses at the end of each encoding line are gradient spoilers that dephase transverse magnetization. **WE**

393. (c) The contrast depends of the TR also, however at low TE times transverse magnetization is still in phase so proton density is high. **WO**

394. (c) Both FOV and the number of slices increase the slab, the acquisition, and the overall SNR for 3D sequences. **WO**

395. (c) The null point is the place where the relaxation curve intersects the transverse plane and where there is no net longitudinal magnetization. **WO**

396. (c) Fast GRE sequences start with a 180° RF pulse, followed by an alternating succession of alpha or partial flip angles followed by the collection of echoes, which is the data acquisition window. **WO**

397. (b) Niobium and titanium are used as the magnetic windings in superconductive magnets. **WE**

398. (b) Paramagnetism, diamagnetism, and ferromagnetism all are terms that describe a substance's response to a magnetic field. **WO**

399. (c) Faraday's law of induction states that a changing magnetic field generates a voltage and current in a conductor. **WO**

400. (b) Magnesium is not a paramagnetic substance. **WO**

401. (c) Zinc and gold are diamagnetic. **WO**

402. (b) B is the magnetic field and H_0 is the magnetic intensity. If "x" has a value of zero or less, the overall magnetic field is zero or less. It is only when "x" is greater than zero that positive magnetic field results. **LU**

403. (d) One G is the strength of the magnetic field measured one centimeter from a straight wire carrying five amps of current. (YO)

404. (d) Superconductive and air-core resistive magnet types require solenoidal magnet designs requiring that the magnetic field produced run horizontally. **LU**

405. (c) The degree of resistance along a wire is determined by Ohm's law. **WE**

406. (b) Niobium titanium becomes superconductive below approximately 10° K. **WE**

407. (b) A greater homogeneity of one ppm is required for spectroscopy, which provides greater tissue specificity. **WE**

408. (d) The magnetic field strength is proportional to the amount of current passed through the loops of wires, the number and size of each loop, and how closely spaced the loops of wires are. **WE**

409. (b) The power of current that generates the gradient strength determines the slope of the gradient. **WE**

410. (c) Only transverse magnetization is received into the RF receiver because of the placement of the receive coil (in the transverse plane) and its relation to the static magnetic field. **LU**

411. (d) The bulk magnetic properties of a substance principally result from electrons. Magnetic susceptibility of a substance is dominated by electronic (electrons) effects. **EL**

412. (b) Iron core magnets create a vertical field requiring solenoidal RF coils. **LU**

413. (b) The orbital angular momentum of the electron is much greater than the dipole generated by the nucleus. Although the MR resonance is based on the nucleus, the magnetic environment is based on the paired or unpaired electrons. **LU**

414. (b) Saddle-shaped coils must be used with horizontal magnetic fields as used in air-core and superconducting magnets. **LU**

415. (c) Phased array coils are individual receive coils for surface imaging and are combined for improved SNR and increased coverage. **WE**

416. (c) The rate of planar surface coil signal drop-off depends on the coil dimension. Very little useful signal is present beyond one radius from the center of the coil ($1/r^2$). **LU**

417. (d) The "Q" of the coil determines the quality factor of the coil based on the patient load and is dependent

on the direct current resistivity of the coil material, the RF resistivity of the coil material, and the coil loading by the patient. **LU**

418. (c) The center frequency lets the scanner know exactly what frequency at which the protons are resonating at the center of the magnet. **EL**

419. (c) During prescan, the transmit and receive coil is tuned, the center frequency is set, and the amount of transmit and receive amplification is determined. **EL**

420. (b) Since another set of coils is used by quadrature coils, that will increase the SNR potential by the square root of the change or the square root of 2. **EL**

421. (b) These terms are arbitrary. They refer to the components of the total signal that are phase shifted 0° and 90° compared with the reference RF oscillator within the scanner. **EL**

422. (a) The RF power adjusts the voltage and current. The amount will determine the actual flip angle of the RF. **EL**

423. (b) The impedance of the transmit/receive coil must be matched to the impedance of the transmission line. If not, a large fraction of the RF power will be reflected by at the coil-transmission line interface. **EL**

424. (d) Since phased array coils have individual receive coils and channels, all of the factors are benefits that increase SNR, coverage, and uniformity. **WE**

425. (c) There are separate receive channels for each coil. **WE**

426. (b) Permanent magnets produce vertical fields requiring solenoidal-type RF coils. **WO**

427. (a) Gradients impose a magnetic gradient over the static magnetic field and will cause an increase in magnetic field on one side of isocenter and a decrease on the other side, creating a graduation of the magnetic field from one end to the other. **WE**

428. (b) Steeper gradients reduce the partial voluming effect, therefore minimizing chemical shift misregistration. Steeper gradients also minimize inhomogeneities in the magnetic fields. **LU**

429. (b) Cross-talk is often the result of nonrectangular RF pulse waveforms. In this situation gaps are recommended. **EL**

430. (c) Gradient magnetic fields are measured based on their field strength per unit of distance — millitesla per meter or mT/m. **EL**

431. (d) Increasing the amplitude of the slice select gradient would create a steeper gradient. Increasing the strength of the gradient while maintaining bandwidth will cause a decrease in slice thickness. **WE**

432. (b) The frequency-selective or "fat sat" method uses a short duration, frequency-selective 90° RF pulse to flip fat magnetization into the transverse plane. While in the transverse plane, fat magnetization is dephased by application of a spoiler gradient. **EL**

433. (b) The phase encoding process is designed to create phase dispersions to identify the location of the MR signal within the matrix. **WO**

434. (c) The slice select gradient is turned on during the time that RF is being applied to the individual slices. This occurs during the 90° and 180° RF pulses **WO**

435. (b) The gradient rise time determines the amount of time or speed necessary to reach full gradient amplitude. **EL**

436. (b) The maximum gradient amplitude of clinical scanners is 10 mT/m. For echo planar and fast imaging, higher amplitudes are sought. **EL**

437. (c) Steep gradients alter the magnetic field more than shallow gradients. **WE**

438. (c) Sagittal slices require that the x-gradient be used for slice selection. **WE**

439. (b) Combined gradient amplitudes are used to create scans off-orthogonally or obliquely. **WE**

440. (b) The z-gradient is used for slice selection, the x-gradient for frequency encoding, leaving the y-gradient for phase encoding. **WE**

441. (c) The higher the magnetic field, the higher the precessional frequency. Protons that experience increas-

ing gradient fields accelerate as they traverse the gradient fields. **WE**

442. (c) The receive coil is placed perpendicular or transverse to the static magnetic field. The signal received, is that of transverse magnetization. **WO**

443. (c) Precession refers to the type of motion that protons spinning on their own axis experience when in the presence of an external magnetic field. **WO**

444. (b) 21.29 mHz. Use the Larmor equation to figure the precessional frequency: Precessional frequency = gyromagnetic ratio x magnetic field. **WE**

445. (a) As the magnetic field changes, the precessional frequencies changes by the same factor. **WE**

446. (b) The earth's magnetic field or force is not strong enough to cause net magnetization of the body's spins. **WE**

447. (a) 10 kG = 10,000 G = 1 T. **WE**

448. (c) A vector has magnitude (amount) and direction. **WO**

449. (b) The Larmor equation states that the precessional frequency is equal to the gyromagnetic moment times the applied magnetic field. **WE**

450. (b) Options one and three are variations of the same formula and represent the Larmor equation. Option number two does not represent the Larmor equation. **WE**

451. (d) The force of attraction of an object exposed to a magnetic field depends on mass, ferromagnetic properties, and rate of change in the field strength. **WE**

452. (c) In a magnetic field there is a tendency for slightly more than half of the net spins to align with the magnetic field or in the ground state. **LU**

453. (d) Proton density reflects only a subset of all protons in fat and water molecules (mobile hydrogen). **LU,PA**

454. (a) Because of the electron cloud that surrounds fat and water and because the electron cloud that surrounds fat is stronger than water, fat is shielded slightly more from the static magnetic field, causing it to

have a slower precessional frequency than water. **WO**

455. (a) One. The atomic number is the number of protons in the nucleus. **WE**

456. (b) Small molecules like water have a much higher rate of molecular motion than the Larmor frequency for any of the current MR instruments. They are, therefore, inefficient at returning energy to the lattice and have long T1 relaxation times. **LU**

457. (c) A dipole-dipole interaction refers to the magnetic interaction between two protons or a proton and an electron. **EL**

458. (b) The act of resonating requires absorbing and re-emitting energy with the same frequency. **EL**

459. (c) Gradient magnetic fields create varying magnetic field strengths whose force proportionately changes the precessional frequencies of the protons within those magnetic fields. **WE**

460. (d) A resonating frequency must be applied perpendicular to the static magnetic field with enough power to tip the net magnetization out of the longitudinal plane. **WE**

461. (b) Use the Larmor equation: 42.58 mHz/T x .64 T = 2.725 mHz. **WE**

462. (d) After a 360° rotation, the wave function can be shown to be identical to that existing at 0°, but with a reversal in its sign. An additional 360° rotation (720° total) is required to return the system to its original state. **EL**

463. (b) The optimal flip angle is 90° only when TR > T1. For sequences in which no transverse steady state is established, MR signal is maximized at the Ernst angle. **EL**

464. (d) An MR signal requires the application of repetitive pulses that have a tendency to reduce the size of the steady state longitudinal magnetization that is flipped to create the MR signal. Although 90° pulses tip the largest fraction of magnetization into the transverse plane, they also reduce transverse magnetization, and overall MR signal may not be

maximized. Therefore a series of partial flip angle pulses may generate a stronger signal than is generated by a series of 90° pulses. **EL**

465. (c) With one single RF pulse there is no steady state. A 90° RF pulse maximizes the most signal return. **EL**

466. (b) RF spoiling is accomplished by semi-randomly changing the phase of the RF carrier from view to view; it does not generate eddy currents, and it is spatially invariant. **EL**

467. (d) The range of RFs in the RF pulse is transmit bandwidth. **WE**

468. (b) The gyromagnetic ratio of hydrogen is 42.5759 mHz per 1 T. **LU**

469. (d) The more frequency the gradients turn on, the more likelihood of increased eddy currents. The longer the sequence or TR, the more time to dissipate the residual field once turned off. **WO**

470. (b) Angular momentum is due to net spin. Net spin occurs when there is an odd number of protons, neutrons, or both in the nucleus. **LU**

471. (d) Molecular motion is dependent on the molecular size, the protein binding, and how efficiently the energy is distributed back to the lattice. **LU**

472. (d) To reach 98% of the full T1 relaxation requires four times the T1 of the tissue or 3200 msec. **WO**

473. (b) By definition, the length of time it takes the spin system to lose phase coherence is based on an exponential relaxation curve. 1T2 is equal to a loss of 63% of net transverse magnetization. **WO**

474. (a) T1 relaxation hastens with Brownian motion therefore thermal relaxation is sometimes used to describe spin-lattice relaxation. **WO**

475. (c) Quadrature coils are much more efficient in the transfer of RF power to the patient, reducing the specific absorption rate requirements by one half compared with linearly polarized coils. **EL**

476. (b) T2 relaxation times do not change primarily with field strength. **WE**

477. (c) Larger molecules such as long-chain fatty acids tumble at frequencies well below the resonant fre-

quency. However rotation of terminal fatty acid groups at higher frequencies allows efficient T1 relaxation. **LU**

478. (d) Pure fluids, like water, tend to have a high rate of molecular motion and thus long T1 relaxation times due to inefficient energy transfer to the lattice. The high frequencies tend to average out the intrinsic field to zero so that the magnetic field is determined by that of the external field, and spin phase is maintained for a longer period of time (long T2). **LU**

479. (b) When the net magnetization is initially flipped into the transverse plane, the maximum transverse magnetization exists. **LU**

480. (c) Circularly polarized or quadrature coil designs have the advantage of detecting more accurately the true position of the magnetization in space because there are two receivers present. Since two separate signals are being recorded, there is a potential SNR gain of $\sqrt{2}$ possible with quadrature coil arrangement. **EL**

481. (c) 1T1 is 63% of regrowth of longitudinal magnetization. **WO**

482. (a) Spin-spin relaxation refers to the transfer of energy from one spinning proton to another during T2 relaxation. **WO**

483. (d) All of these flow effects exhibit increased signal intensity. **LU**

484. (a) Fat. The T1 growth curve indicates that over a period of time fat will relaxes faster, regrowing longitudinal magnetization faster. **WO**

485. (c) The T2 relaxation of cerebral spinal fluid is approximately 300 msec. This is very long and therefore is bright on most if not all T2-weighted images. **WO**

486. (b) Bulk magnetic properties of a substance principally result from electrons, whereas the NMR phenomenon involves nuclei (protons and neutrons). **EL**

487. (a) The RF pulse (B_1) is applied perpendicular to the static magnetic field for maximum RF absorption. **WO**

488. (d) Gradient coils function to provide linearly distorted spatial variations in the magnetic field, altering precessional frequencies for spatial encoding. **WE**

489. (c) The gradient slope and the transmit bandwidth determine the slice thickness. **WE**

490. (a) 1 G/cm = 0.1 mT/m. **WO**

491. (b) 10 G/cm means that the local magnetic field increases by 5 G at one end of a 1 meter gradient coil, and decreases it by 5 G at the other. **WO**

492. (b) The slice select gradient is applied when RF needs to be transmitted into the selected slices or slab, which is during the 90° and 180° RF pulses. **WO**

493. (a) Transaxial slices are created with a gradient that graduates the magnetic field from superior to inferior in relation to patient orientation. **WE**

494. (b) Oblique images are created using two sets of slice select gradients to determine slice. **WE**

495. (b) Phase encoding is usually performed after the initial RF pulse has been applied and before refocusing net transverse magnetization. **LU**

496. (b) The y-gradient graduates the magnetic field from anterior to posterior creating coronal slices. **WE**

497. (c) Oblique images angled between sagittal and transaxial require x- and y-gradient simultaneous amplification to graduate the magnetic field, stimulating oblique image slices. **WE**

498. (d) K-space is a holding place for the raw data or time domain data. **WE**

499. (d) Rows near the center of k-space correspond to data collected with low amplitude or low order phase encoding gradients. Rows near the top of k-space correspond to data acquired with high-amplitude or high-order phase encoding gradients, producing high spatial resolution and low signal amplitude. **WE**

500. (b) The frequency encoding gradient is also turned on during the phase encoding process to assure that there are no phase dispersions due to the frequency–encoding process during the collection of the echo. **WO**

501. (d) Only on the central reference lines in both direction are the magnetic moments both in phase and at the maximum signal amplitude. **WE**

502. (c) The term chemical shift refers to the difference in resonant frequency of protons due to local differences in chemical environment. **WO**

503. (b) Aliasing or wraparound results when the receive frequency range is insufficient to assign all the returned MR signals during phase and frequency encoding. If the FOV is too small for the area of interest, there is ambiguous assignment of the MR signals, resulting in aliasing. **WO**

504. (c) Motion can occur in all directions, however, it will be displayed in the phase-encoding direction. During phase-encoding there is a change in gradient amplitude before each slice is acquired. If flow or motion occurs, it results in the misassignment in k-space during the acquisition. **WO**

505. (c) The zebra stripes-like artifact appears from the misassignment of frequencies in the phase-encoding direction (aliasing) and when acquiring a GRE sequence and an FOV too small for the area of interest. **WO**

506. (a) Truncation artifacts appear as repetitious bright and dark bands and occur at the interface of very high and very low signal transitions. **WO**

507. (b) 149.03. Multiply 3.5 ppm x the precessional frequency at 1.0T (42.58 mHz/T). **WO**

508. (c) Water will have a higher precessional frequency than fat. The electron cloud that surrounds water does not shield the nucleus as much as the cloud surrounding fat's nucleus. The effect from the magnetic field will be stronger on water, increasing its precessional frequency. **WO**

509. (d) Most electrical components, if powered and not shielded, can cause RF interference during scanning. **WO**

510. (d) FID artifacts appear like a "zipper" across the center of the image, although manufacturers now have shifted the artifact to the edge of the image. FID ar-

tifacts are caused by remnant FID that remain after the 180° RF pulse. **WO**

511. (b) Gibb's artifact. The initial overshoot on either side of the interface (sine wave) persists with an amplitude of 9% of the step function height. **WO**

512. (c) With a 1.5T magnetic field the chemical shift is 224 Hz. If the total receive bandwidth is 32 kHz, then there is a 7 pixel shift due to chemical shift. **WO**

513. (b) Frequency aliasing. The Nyquist theorem states that the signal must be sampled a minimum of twice per cycle. If not, peaks and valleys of different frequencies can resemble one another when Fourier transformed, creating frequency aliasing. **WO**

514. (c) Oversampling (antialiasing) assigns addresses to frequencies outside the FOV. Steep bandpass filters also filter frequencies outside the FOV. **WO**

515. (c) Light bulbs can cause RF discreets and herringbone due to RF emissions that are not part of the scanning transmit or receive bandwidths. **WO**

516. (b) a Gradient moment nulling is a flow compensation technique used to compensate for flowing spins. Gradients are used to rephase and dephase spins that flow into the region of interest. **WO**

517. (d) The aorta is pulsating during the image process causing motion replication in the phase encoding direction. **WO**

518. (d) In the frequency direction, chemical shift appears as a low signal intensity on the high-frequency side and a high signal intensity on the low-frequency side of the organ. **WO**

519. (c) Truncation artifacts appear at the interface of low and high intensity signal transitions such as cortical bone and bone marrow. **WO**

520. (b) SNR is proportional to the square root of NEX and to the voxel volume. The SNR is proportional to the square root of the number of phase encode steps. **WE**

521. (d) Increasing the matrix step and decreasing the pixel size reduces partial voluming while increasing spatial resolution. **WO**

522. (d) To maintain SNR, the number of acquisitions must increase fourfold to compensate for the 50% reduction in slice thickness. **WE**

523. (d) All three are capable of inducing eddy currents. **EL**

524. (c) Decreases in slice thickness reduce the area scanned per slice, reducing SNR and partial voluming. Reducing partial voluming increases spatial resolution. **WE**

525. (a) CSE pulse sequences use 180° RF pulses to minimize magnetic field inhomogeneities that cause T2 dephasing. **WO**

Post Test Answers

1. (d) All of the listed implants are contraindicated for MRI scanning. **WE**
2. (d) The magnetic field may cause changes in the pacemaker programming or induce a current in the lead wire that could cause burns to the patient. **WE**
3. (b) A hand-held magnet is an acceptible procedure for checking for ferrous qualities in accessory devices. **WE**
4. (c) Anaphylactoid reactions involve respiratory, cardiovascular, cutaneous, or gastrointestinal distress. **SH**
5. (d) The orientation of the gradient field, the patient's size, and the frequency of the stimulus are all factors that may induce a physiologic response to induced voltage during scanning. **SH**
6. (a) Magnetophosphenes are visual sensations which have been reported after patients have been in the gradient magnetic field. **SH**
7. (d) The FDA has stated that the safe SAR level for the head is 3.2 W per kg. **SH**
8. (b) The newer, fast sequences have increased RF deposition compared with conventional spin echo sequences. **SH**
9. (b) Since respiratory depression is the most common reaction to sedation, anesthesiologists consider the use of the pulse oximeter to be a standard practice for monitoring sedated or anesthetized patients. **SH**
10. (b) Paramagnetic contrast agents decrease both the T1 and T2 relaxation times of tissue. **SH**
11. (a) Magnevist is an ionic compound. **SH**
12. (a) Patients with asthma or allergic respiratory disorders are most likely to develop serious reactions to contrast. **SH**
13. (c) The coronal projection best displays the collateral ligaments. **BU**
14. (c) Increased SNR is the biggest advantage to using a surface coil. **WO**
15. (a) Reduced RF deposition reduces the SAR to the patient. **WO**

16. (c) The TMJ is a receive only coil. **WO**

17. (b) "A basic rule of thumb when using surface coil is to match the FOV to the size of the coil. In the example, the 5" circular coil gave less SNR since the coil was larger than the FOV. Signal outside the FOV aliased into the FOV, causing decreased SNR." The 3" surface coil is best for the TMJ. **WO**

18. (d) The phased array coil gives high SNR and covers a large area. **WO**

19. (a) A Helmholtz configuration is considered a volume coil. **WO**

20. (b) Negative contrast enhancement occurs when the tissue of interest appears darker on images following ferromagnetic or superparamagnetic contrast. **WO**

21. (a) Divide the 75 pounds by 2.2 (lb per kg), then multiply the kilograms by .2 mL/kg = 6 cc. **WE**

22. (c) The maximum dose is 20 ml or cc. **WE, MO, OM, PR**

23. (d) Patients with sickle cell may develop sickle cell crisis after the injection of gadolinium. Since the contrast filters out through the kidneys and liver, it is often contraindicated to administer contrast to patients in renal failure. Contrast is contraindicated for pregnant patients since it would be impossible to help a fetus if it developed a reaction. **WE**

24. (d) The choroid plexus and pineal and pituitary glands all routinely enhance after the administration of contrast. **WE**

25. (d) The matrix 256 x 256 provides high resolution, but low SNR. **WE**

26. (a) Maximum intensity projection (MIP) creates a 2D projective image from the brightest pixel on a 3D dataset. **BU**

27. (c) Gadolinium is a paramagnetic product. **BU**

28. (c) Oral contrast is dark on T1 and dark on T2. **BU**

29. (d) It is important to remember that a surface coil gives a restricted FOV, therefore, positioning is critical. If the coil is not perpendicular to the X/Y plane, a significant reduction in SNR results. **BU**

30. (a) Hemosiderin is dark on both T1- and T2-weighted images. **ST**

31. (a) The transverse and coronal planes have become widely accepted as the planes of choice when viewing the orbit. **BU**

32. (c) The petrous bone and mastoid air cells are black on imges because of the low signal from dense bone and air. **BU**

33. (a) Major white matter tracts are best demonstrated on the axial plane when imaging the brain. **BU**

34. (d) EPI is an extremely fast method of acquiring an image from one selective excitation pulse. **BU**

35. (a) Compared to the other stated veins, the hepatic vein is most superior in orientation. **MO**

36. (b) The portal vein drains into the inferior mesenteric vein, the superior mesenteric vein, and the splenic vein. **AP**

37. (c) The coverage of a coil is 1/2 the radius. **ST**

38. (c) Gradient moment nulling (flow compensation) makes vessels appear bright. **WE**

39. (a) Time of flight (TOF) relies on flow-related enhancement to distinguish moving spins from stationary tissue. **WE**

40. (c) "TOF-MRA is sensitive to flow coming into the FOV, and spins with slow flow can be saturated in volume imaging. For this reason, 3D TOF should be used in areas of high velocity flow (intra-cranial applications), and 2D TOF in areas of slower velocity flow (carotids, peripheral vessels, and the venous systems." **WE**

41. (a) Phase contrast imaging uses velocity differences or phase shifts to provide image contrast in flowing vessels. **WE**

42. (a) Cine is a technique that collects data continuously through the cardiac cycle. **WE**

43. (b) The Circle of Willis is best demonstrated with the 3D TOF. **SI**

44. (a) The carotid arteries are best demonstrated on the 2D TOF sequences. **SI**

45. (b) Cine is performed during a gradient echo sequence. **WE**

46. (c) EPI is currently the fastest of the high-speed MRI techniques. **ST**

47. (b) Laminar flow is faster at the center of the vessel than at the vessel wall. **WE**

48. (c) Turbulent flow has different velocities which change erratically, and fluctuate randomly. **WE**

49. (d) TOF effects depend on the velocity of flow, the echo time, and the slice thickness. **WE**

50. (d) Flow related enhancement occurs when the flow decreases, allowing a larger number of nuclei to be present for the 90° and the 180° RF pulses. **WE**

51. (c) Structure 1 in Figure 33 is the anterior cerebral artery. **OS**

    (Key to Figure 33: 1. Anterior cerebral artery; 2. Middle cerebral artery; 3.Posterior cerebral artery.)

52. (c) Structure 2 in Figure 33 is the middle cerebral artery. **OS**

53. (b) Structure 2 in Figure 34 is the middle cerebral artery. **OS**

    (Key to Figure 34: 1. Anterior cerebral artery; 2. Middle cerebral artery; 3. Anterior communicating artery; 4.Posterior communicating artery.)

54. (c) Structure 3 in Figure 34 is the anterior communicating artery. **OS**

55. (a) Structure 1 in Figure 35 is the internal carotid artery. **OS**

    (Key to Figure 35: 1. Internal carotid artery; 2. External carotid artery; 3. Common carotid artery: 4. Vertebral artery.)

56. (b) Structure 3 in Figure 35 is the common carotid artery. **OS**

57. (b) Structure 4 in Figure 35 is the vertebral artery. **OS**

58. (d) On a sagittal projection, the bladder is directly anterior to the uterus. **AP**

59. (c) Structure 1 in Figure 36 is the stomach. **BA**

(Key to Figure 36: 1. Stomach; 2. Pancreas;
3. Aorta; 4. Vena cava; 5. Portal vein; 6. Right Kid-
ney; 8. Liver; 9. Bowel.)

60. (b) Structure 2 in Figure 36 is the pancreas. **BA**
61. (a) Structure 3 in Figure 36 is the aorta. **BA**
62. (a) Structure 4 in Figure 36 is the inferior vena cava. **BA**
63. (b) Structure 9 in Figure 36 is the bowel. **BA**
64. (c) Structure 8 in Figure 36 is the liver. **BA**
65. (a) In order to display the veins only in a vascular study in the femoral area, saturation pulses should be placed superiorly to saturate out the arteries.
66. (a) In order to display the carotid arteries, it is neccessary to place saturation pulses superiorly to saturate the veins that are draining down, back to the heart.
67. (b) The axial projection of the orbit in example 37 was acquired with the spin echo pulse sequence, post contrast, using fat saturation. (Note the accumulation of contrast in the lateral ventricle.) **BU**

(Key to Figure 37: 1. Orbital globe; 2. Cerebral
peduncle; 3. Cerebral aqueduct; 4. Sphenoid sinus;
5. Lateral rectus muscle; 5. Temporal lobe.)

68. (a) Structure 4 in Figure 37 is the sphenoid sinus. **BU**
69. (c) A Wilm's tumor is a rapidly developing tumor of the kidney that usually occurs in children. **ST**
70. (c) The superior sagittal sinus and cerebral veins drain down into the jugular vein. **AP**
71. (b) TE is the length of time from the application of the 90° RF pulse to the collection of the spin echo. **WO**
72. (d) The time of inversion, TI, determines the length of time tissues are allowed to relax from the negative z-plane prior to excitation by the 90° RF pulse. **WO**
73. (c) Both GRE and 3DFT GRE pulse sequences employ initial RF pulses of less than 90°. Fast GRE sequences begin with a 180° RF pulse. **WO**
74. (d) The null point is defined as .69T1 of the tissue and is where net magnetization intersects the transverse plane. At the null point there is no net longitudinal magnetization and tissues are suppressed. **WO**

75. (c) Both CSE and FSE sequences are capable of producing true T2-weighted images. **WO**

76. (c) GRE sequences do not use 180° refocusing RF pulses and are unable to reduce the magnetic susceptibility effects caused by inhomogeneities in the magnetic field. **WE**

77. (b) GRE typically use flip angle of less than 90°, although not required. **WO**

78. (d) Conventional double SE sequences with a long TR acquire first echo with a long TR and short TE. The second later echo is acquired with a long TR and a short TE, producing a proton density first echo and a T2-weighted second echo image. **WE**

79. (b) 3DFT images are capable of acquiring a large number of slices. The larger the number of slices needed, the larger the slab initially excited by the RF pulse. This increases SNR at the expense of time. **WO**

80. (b) The ETE, or effective TE, is placed in the center of k-space and contributes most to the contrast of the overall image. **WO**

81. (b) The 180° RF pulse refocuses net transverse magnetization after it starts dephasing once the 90° RF pulse has been terminated. **WO**

82. (d) Partial Fourier technique reduces imaging time by acquiring half the phase encoding steps. For fractional NEX imaging, SNR is reduced by a factor of $\frac{\sqrt{1}}{2}$, approximately 70% compared with a conventional one NEX sequence. **EL**

83. (b) Partial or fractional echo. The frequency encoding gradient is on during the sampling of the echo. Partial sampling of the echo occurs when the frequency encoding gradient gathers part of the returned signal. **WE**

84. (c) At least half of k-space must be filled to produce the image. This process requires "zero filling" the rest of the sample. Partial averaging reduces scan time. **WE**

85. (b) Fourier transform converts time varying MR signals into a spectrum of complex frequencies. **EL**

86. (c) Once the center frequency has been determined, an RF pulse transmits a range of frequencies to excite a slice of a particular slice thickness. **EL**

87. (d) Fractional echo imaging requires that only a portion of the echo is sampled. The echo does not have to be centered on the middle of the frequency encoding gradient. This allows the sampling window to be shifted adjusting where the sampling occurs to maximize signal and acquiring shorter TE times. **WE**

88. (c) If the bandwidth is constant, adjusting the slice thickness requires the gradient slope or strength be adjusted. **EL**

89. (d) TOF MRA sequences use gradient moment nulling techniques to refocus flowing spins for higher signal return and vessel enhancement. Very short TEs and moderate flip angles are used to enhance the returned signal of flowing spins within the vessel and to separate them from stationary spins. **EL**

90. (b) PC MRA activate bipolar gradients to distinguish stationary spins that experience no net phase shift from moving spins. Moving spins with a constant velocity experience a phase shift proportional to flow velocity, to the amplitude of the bipolar gradient, and to the time interval between the gradient lobes. **EL**

91. (c) Maximum enhancement of flow occurs when the vessel is perpendicular to the plane of imaging. TOF techniques are thus somewhat insensitive to in-plane flow. **EL**

92. (c) Velocity encoding, VENC, is measured in centimeters per second (cm/sec). **EL**

93. (d) Spins moving with a constant velocity experience a phase shift proportional to flow velocity, to the amplitude of the bipolar gradient and to the time interval between the gradient lobes. **EL**

94. (a) TOF sequences are most useful for acquiring relatively rapid flow in vessels that pass perpendicular

to the imaging plane (e.g., aorta, iliac, femoral and carotid arteries). **EL**

95. (a) Short TR enhances T1 contrast and short TE minimizes the T2 contrast effect while providing proton density signal. **WO**

96. (c) K-space stores raw data into files converted to signal intensities or processed domain. **WE**

97. (b) The central lines of k-space are filled with low amplitude phase encoding gradients that return high SNR. The effective TE is placed in the central lines of k-space with similar echoes in adjacent k-space lines. **WE**

98. (b) Matrix size affects spatial resolution and SNR but does not directly affect contrast. **WO**

99. (d) Long TR, short TE sequences create images with high proton concentration. Long TR sequences allow more complete T1 regrowth. Short TE times do not allow significant dephasing of transverse magnetization. This combination creates PD-weighted image contrast. **WO**

100. (c) Oversampling in the frequency encoding direction provides more samples, increasing SNR and spatial resolution, while also limiting frequency aliasing. **WE**

101. (c) Phase encoding requires multiple encoding steps that use varying gradient amplitudes that can cause motion to appear if the tissue or spins move or flow during the acquisition. Phase encoding perpendicular to flow is recommended and to the short axis of the patient to reduce artifacts. **WE**

102. (b) Increasing TR provides more time to acquire slices. The last echo collected determines the amount of time remaining "dead time," or time delay before another RF pulse is required. During this dead time, more slices can be acquired. The more time available, based on TR/TE, the more slices can be acquired. **WO**

103. (b) $(NEX)^2$ is directly proportional to SNR. Decrease in NEX decreases SNR. **WE**

104. (b) An increase in phase encoding while holding FOV constant requires smaller pixels. Spatial resolution increases and scan time is proportional to the number of phase steps. **WE**

105. (c) TI determines how much longitudinal relaxation occurs from the negative z-plane prior to excitation with the 90° RF pulse. This, in turn, defines the area of T1 regrowth as signal is returned to create the MR image. **WO**

106. (c) STIR sequences suppress the signal from tissues that have relatively short T1 times such as fat and gadolinium enhancing lesions. **WO**

107. (c) Reducing the TE time does not allow significant dephasing of the transverse magnetization. Since the spins in the transverse plane are still in phase, the in-phase protons return a large signal and proton concentration increases. **WO**

108. (b) Pixel size = FOV/matrix size;
FOV = matrix x pixel size. **WE**

109. (b) SNR is proportional to voxel size, which is matrix size and slice thickness. **WE**

110. (b) For shorter scan times and specific contrast, only a portion of the longitudinal magnetization is flipped into the transverse plane in GRE pulse sequences. **WE**

111. (c) An increase in the number of frequency encodings will increase spatial resolution and FOV, therefore reducing frequency aliasing, however the scan time is not affected. **WO**

112. (c) TE controls the amount of time allowed for transverse magnetization to decay before collecting the echo. **WE**

113. (d) The number of excitations, averages, and acquisitions are interchangeable terms that represent the number of times data is collected with the same amplitude of the phase encoding gradient. **EL**

114. (b) $\sqrt{2}$; SNR $= \sqrt{NEX}$ **WE**

115. (a) Reducing noise while maintaining signal is challenging. A way to reduce noise is to reduce the re-

ceive bandwidth. As less noise is sampled as a proportion of signal, the SNR increases. **WE**

116. (b) Matrix is composed of phase-encoding and frequency encoding steps. The steps are comprised of pixels. The size and number of pixels and steps determine FOV. **WE**

117. (d) Reducing the pixel size, FOV, and slice thickness cause a reduction in partial voluming. **WE**

118. (c) Doubling FOV requires doubling the area or voxel volume in both axes quadrupling the SNR. **WE**

119. (a) The number of slices allowed per TR, depends on the length of time for the last TE to be acquired (duty cycle). The shorter the TE the more time available to acquire additional slices. **WO**

120. (b) Rectangular FOV. Sampling alternate phase encode lines in k-space while leaving the maximum and minimum amplitudes of the phase encoding gradient unchanged halves the number of phase encoding steps and doubles the increment between successive steps. This creates a rectangular FOV. **EL**

121. (d) GRE pulse sequences are very susceptible to motion. **WE**

122. (d) All of the parameters affect SNR in the proportions listed. **WE**

123. (d) Symmetrical and isotropic voxels resolve the highest detail when data is reconstructed into other planes. **WE**

124. (b) Volume images are acquired using shallow gradients that yield high amplitude signals, increasing SNR. **WE**

125. (c) Echo train spacing is the distance between successive echoes collected during each TR. **EL**

126. (b) Slice thickness, phase encode steps, and flip angle increase the amount of signal collected and the SNR. **WE**

127. (b) The SNR of 3D volume images would decrease if the FOV, the number of slices, and the TR are reduced. **WE**

128. (b) Increasing TR, decreasing TE, and reducing the receive bandwidth allow for higher proton density and stronger MR signal increasing SNR. **WE**

129. (c) Slice thickness, FOV and matrix all affect spatial resolution. A reduction in size of the voxel will increase spatial resolution. **WE**

130. (b) 0.625 mm; FOV/matrix = pixel size. **WE**

131. (c) The longer the time to collect the echo, the more T2 dephasing allowed and the lower the SNR. A decrease in signal often presents with image graininess. **WO**

132. (c) Volume elements are termed voxels. **WE**

133. (b) Faraday's law of induction states that a changing magnetic field will generate a voltage and current in a conductor. **EL**

134. (b) Shim coils are used to redistribute the magnetic flux lines to make the magnetic field level or homogeneous. **WE**

135. (d) Superconductive magnets designs are used most frequently in MR imagers. Other designs are also effective. **WE**

136. (b) Superconductive magnet design allows for the generation of high magnetic fields. Permanent and resistive have field strength limits. **LU**

137. (b) Permanent and iron core resistive magnets that produce vertical magnetic fields require solenoidal RF coils. **LU**

138. (b) The bigger the coil, the larger the available FOV. As FOV increases, SNR decreases. **LU**

139. (b) RF pulses are energy bursts transmitted at the resonant frequency of hydrogen used to excite the nucleus. **WE**

140. (b) RF must be applied perpendicular to the static magnetic field to transmit the RF power fully to the patient. If the RF is not applied perpendicular to B_0, the transmitted RF can add magnetism to the static field, a termed called coupling. Coupling renders the RF pulse less effective. **WE**

141. (c) Gradient amplifiers provide power and amplification to the gradients. **WE**

142. (c) Ferromagnetic substances that come into contact with magnetic fields result in strong attraction and alignment. They retain magnetization even when the external magnetic field has been removed. **WE**

143. (b) The magnetic susceptibility of a substance is the ability of external magnetic fields to affect the nuclei of a particular atom and is related to the electron configuration of that atom. **WE**

144. (c) RF pulses are secondary oscillating magnetic fields formed as a result of passing a current through a RF receive coil. **WE**

145. (b) Transmit bandwidth is a range of frequencies transmitted to excite a slice thickness. **WE**

146. (b) The slope of the slice select gradient and the slice thickness determine the slice gap required. **WE**

147. (b) Stimulated echo occur from the action of three or more unequally spaced RF pulses. The echoes result from the presence of longitudinal magnetization that has been stored along the z-axis by the second RF pulse. **EL**

148. (d) Precession is the wobbling motion that the nucleus experiences when it is subjected to an external magnetic field. The nucleus spins on its own axis as well as about the magnetic field. **WO**

149. (b) Using the Larmor equation the precessional frequency of hydrogen exposed to a 1.9 T magnetic field is 80.9 mHz. **WE**

150. (d) The equilibrium state exists when atoms are precessing in the direction of the static magnetic field and are out of phase and are fully relaxed. **WO**

151. (c) Net magnetic vector describes the amount or strength of the net spins and the direction of the spins. **WE**

152. (b) Resonance occurs when transmitted energy matches the frequency and oscillation of atoms precessing in a magnetic field. Resonance is the absorption and re-emission of energy. **WE**

153. (c) Flip angle. The amount and duration of the RF pulse determines how far the longitudinal magnetization is tipped. **EL**

154. (d) Voltage is induced in the receive coil when the net magnetic vector precesses at the Larmor frequency in the transverse plane. **WE**

155. (b) As the magnitude of transverse magnetization decreases, so does the magnitude of the voltage induced in the receiver coil. This is free induction decay (FID). **WE**

156. (c) T2 relaxation results from the magnetic interaction of neighboring spins as they precess in phase and begin to exchange energies while in the transverse plane. **WE**

157. (d) Extended sampling time and variable bandwidth, interchangeable terms, are used to increase SNR by extending the sampling window while reducing the bandwidth during image acquisition. **EL**

158. (d) All of the terms represent the technique of adding additional gradient lobes before signal readout to compensate for motion. **EL**

159. (a) 3.2 minutes. In FSE sequences, the scan time is divided by the number of echo trains or ETL. **WE**

160. (b) Because of the placement and interaction of the return signal and the receive coil, only transverse magnetization can be measured directly. **LU**

161. (b) The signal within the entire voxel volume is averaged to determine the signal intensity that represents the range of signals within the voxel. **LU**

162. (c) The x-gradient imposes a linearly distorted gradient magnetic field over the static magnetic field, varying the field from left to right. **LU**

163. (b) Time domain represents the MR signal plotted as amplitude vs. time. **LU**

164. (b) Spin phase effects refer to changes in precession angle that protons undergo when they move within a magnetic field gradient. **EL**

165. (b) 2DFT spatial encoding has three main processes: slice-selection, phase encoding, and frequency encoding. **LU**

166. (a) Frequency encoding is performed during the readout of the echo and creates a one-to-one correspondence between the frequency of the returned signal

and the source's position along the readout direction. **LU**

167. (c) T1-dependent suppression is acquired using STIR. **EL**

168. (b) Unsaturated flowing spins experience an excitation pulse, producing a large transverse magnetization. This magnetization returns a large signal called entry phenomenon, that is proportional to slice thickness and repetition time. **WO**

169. (c) Even-echo rephasing occurs when the signal from laminar flow is rephased and collected in symmetrical echoes. In the first echo laminar flow is dephased, resulting in low signal return. The second echo acquires rephased laminar flow signal and presents as a bright signal intensity. The echoes must be spaced evenly for this phenomenon to occur. **WO**

170. (b) Aliasing occurs when the assignment of frequencies from the MR signal is ambiguous, causing signals with different frequencies but similar phase or frequencies to be placed in the same location. **WO**

171. (a) The electron cloud surrounding fat and water's nucleus shields the nucleus from the magnetic field to some degree. This causes fat and water precessional frequencies to be similar. Fourier transform places them in the incorrect location, causing a misassignment and shifting of frequencies. **WO**

172. (c) The precessional frequency of hydrogen in a 1.5 T magnetic field is 63.8 mHz. To determine the chemical shift of fat and water multiply 63.8 mHz by 3.5 ppm, which will equal 224 Hz. **WO**

173. (b) Gibb's artifact is similar in appearance to truncation artifact. Gibb's artifact is caused by the first peak of the sine wave adjacent to the high contrast interface to always overshoot the ideal intensity line. **WO**

174. (c) B1 is the RF (oscillating secondary magnetic field) applied and is produced by the RF transmit coil. **WO**

175. (c) Paramagnetic substances, such as gadolinium, align with the direction of the magnetic field, their mag-

netic moments adding together. This causes a disruption in the local homogeneity within the tissues, shortening T1 and T2 relaxation. **WO**

References

AP   Applegate E: The Sectional Anatomy Learning System, Philadelphia, WB Saunders, 1991.

BA   Barrett C, Anderson L ,Holder L, Poliakoff S: Primer of Sectional Anatomy with MRI and CT Correlation. Baltimore, Williams and Wilkins, 1994.

BR   Brasch R: MRI Contrast Enhancement in the Central Nervous System, New York, Raven Press, 1993.

BU   Bushong S: Magnetic Resonance Imaging: Physical and Biological Principals. Chicago, Mosby, 1996.

EL   Elster AD: Questions and Answers in Magnetic Resonance Imaging. St. Louis, Mosby, 1994.

KE   Keller P, Drayer B: Signa Applications Guide, Volume 3. Milwaukee, GE Medical Systems, August 1990.

LU   Lufkin RB: The MRI Manual. Chicago, Year Book Medical Publishers, Inc, 1990.

MA   Magnevist Product Insert, Berlex Laboratories, 1990.

MI   Mills R, Ortendahl D, Hylton N, et al: Partial Flip Angle MR Imaging. Radiology 1987; 162: 531–539.

MO   Moller T: Pocket Atlas of Cross Sectional Anatomy: CT and MRI. New York, Thieme Medical Publishers, 1994.

NO   Nolte J: The Human Brain. St. Louis, CV Mosby Company, 1981.

OM   Omniscan Product Insert, Sanofi Winthrop Pharmaceuticals, 1991.

OS   Osborn A: Introduction to Cerebral Angiography. Cambridge, Harper & Row, 1980.

PA   Partain CL, James Jr., AE, Rollo FD: Nuclear Magnetic Resonance (NMR) Imaging. Philadelphia, WB Saunders, 1983.

POTC Potchen EJ, Haacke EM, Siebert JE, Gottschalk A: Magnetic Resonance Angiography. St. Louis, Mosby–Year Book, Inc, 1993.

POTT Potter P, Perry A: Basic Nursing Theory in Practice, 3rd edition. St. Louis, Mosby, 1995.

PR   Prohance Product Insert, Squibb Diagnostics, 1993.

SC   Scherer J, Timby B: Introductory Medicine for Surgical Nursing, 6th edition. Philadelphia, JB Lippincott, 1995.

SH   Shellock F, Kanal E: Magnetic Resonance Bioeffects, Safety, and Patient Management. New York, Raven Press, 1994.

ST   Stark D, Bradley W: Magnetic Resonance Imaging. St. Louis, Mosby Yearbook, 1992.

STO   Stoller D: Magnetic Resonance Imaging in Orthopedic and Sports Medicine. Philadelphia, JB Lippincott 1993.

TH   Thomas C: Taber's Cyclopedic Medical Dictionary. Philadelphia, FA Davis Co., 1985.

WE   Westbrook C, Kaut C: MRI In Practice. Oxford, Blackwell Scientific Publications, 1993.

WO   Woodward P, Freimarck R: MRI for Technologists. New York, McGraw-Hill, 1995.

YO   Young SW: Magnetic Resonance Imaging Basic Principals. New York, Raven Press, 1988.

Symbols and Abbreviations

2D	Two dimensional
3D	Three dimensional
3DFT	3D Fourier Transform
A	Amps
CSE	Conventional Spin Echo
ETL	Echo Train Length
ETS	Echo Train Spacing
FA	Flip Angle
Fast GRE	Fast Gradient Recalled Echo
FID	Free induction decay
FOV	Field of View
FSE	Fast Spin Echo
G	Gauss
G/cm	Gauss per centimeter
GRE	Gradient Recalled Echo
Hz	Hertz
IR	Inversion Recovery
kG	Kilogauss
msec	Milliseconds
mHz	Megahertz
mHz/T	Megahertz per tesla
min	Minutes
MIP	Maximum intensity projection
MR	Magnetic resonance
MRA	Magnetic resonance angiography
mT/m	Millitesla per meter
M_z	Longitudinal magnetization (z-plane)
NEX	Number of excitations, averages, acquisitions
NMR	Nuclear magnetic resonance
Npe	Number of phase encode steps
Nslices	Number of slices
PC	Phase Contrast
PD	Proton Density
ppm	Particles per million
RF	Radiofrequency
SE	Spin Echo
SNR	Signal-to-noise ratio
SSFP	Steady state free precession

STIR	Short TI inversion recovery
T	Tesla
TD	Time delay
TE	Time to echo
TI	Time of inversion
TOF	Time of flight
TR	Time of repetition
V	Volts
VENC	Velocity encoding
W/kg	Watts per kilogram